With the wisdom of the Bible  observant pastor, Simon has g the much longed for or equally can see dreams of freedom boredom. But by thoughtfull helpfully shows how, approached ..... freedom through service.

As an active and reluctant retiree of 5 years I found encouragement as Scriptural reminders of our worth in Christ and God's design of us for freedom in service rather than self-indulgence, a tonic.

The challenges of the book come from an experienced and loving pastor, whose intent to help his readers catch, or rediscover, the joys of trusting and serving Christ clearly shines through. We are not being got at, but lovingly reminded, in very practical ways, that there is real life to be enjoyed in retirement.

Simon's book will be of great value to workers, their families, those approaching and already retired. With expectations vital to any life change, the encouragement to godly and realistic expectations is a great boon. Saving us from unhealthy cul-de-sacs by opening up new vistas for the last lap, is a gift worthy of personal reading and small group attention.

I am very happy to commend Simon's book and thank him for the work he has put in to helping us in this very practical way.

Rt. Rev Dr Peter Brain

Simon challenges us to rethink about the time God has given us on earth, and how we look at retirement against that backdrop. Is retirement from gainful employment really our time to relax, or an opportunity to serve God with that extra time He has given us? A most important discussion.

Rev Dr Stephen Rarig

Distinctively Christian Retirement

A Biblical call to serve Jesus well in older age

Simon van Bruchem

Published by Written for our Instruction

www.writtenforourinstruction.com

Copyright © Simon van Bruchem 2022

The moral right of the author has been asserted in accordance with the Copyright Amendment (Moral Rights) Act 2000.

All rights reserved. Except as permitted under the Australian Copyright Act 1968 (for example, fair dealing for the purposes of study, research, criticism or review) no part of this publication may be reproduced, stored in a retrieval system, or transmitted in any form or by any means, electronic, mechanical, photocopying, recording or otherwise, without the written permission of the publisher.

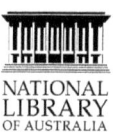 A catalogue record for this work is available from the National Library of Australia

https://www.nla.gov.au/collections

Title:	Distinctively Christian Retirement
Subtitle:	A Biblical call to serve Jesus well in older age
Author:	van Bruchem, Simon (1978–)
ISBNs:	9780648993445 (paperback) 9780648993452 (ebook – epub) 9780648993469 (ebook – mobi)
Subjects:	RELIGION/Christian Living/Social Issues; General; FAMILY & RELATIONSHIPS/Life Stages/Later Years; SELF-HELP/Aging

Cover concept by Simon van Bruchem

Cover layout by Ally Mosher at allymosher.com

Also By Simon van Bruchem

Fear Not: What the Bible has to say about angels, demons, the occult and Satan

For Andrea
*I look forward to continuing to serve Jesus
with you as we grow old together*

Contents

Introduction We believe a lie... 1

Section 1 Retirement is not the paradise we are looking for

Chapter 1 A history lesson: how did we get here? 9

Chapter 2 What makes your life worthwhile?........................... 17

Chapter 3 Doing nothing can kill you; the need for purpose 33

Chapter 4 Death sharpens the mind.. 45

Chapter 5 Don't substitute 'retirement' for 'heaven' 61

Section 2 Regaining a firm foundation: What the Bible says about age and maturity

Chapter 6 Direct Biblical teaching on age and maturity........... 83

Chapter 7 The Biblical example of older believers 95

Chapter 8 Seeking the kingdom first in older age................... 115

Section 3 Practical challenges retirement poses

Chapter 9 Fighting the urge to criticise change and idolise the 'good old days' 131

Chapter 10 Serving Jesus despite loss of energy, disability, and other limitations 145

Section 4 Living out a godly life in retirement

Chapter 11 Retirement and money 161

Chapter 12 Retirees in the church family 175

Chapter 13 Being salt and light as a retiree............................ 189

Closing challenge: An intentionally God-glorifying retirement 201

Acknowledgements... 205

About the Author 206

Endnotes... 207

Introduction
We believe a lie

When we think of retirement, we often think of the glorious time of life where we walk hand in hand with our loved one along a beach or sip champagne on our yacht. According to the superannuation funds' glossy brochures, retirement is a time to finally focus on ourselves. We can do what we want to do, when we want to do it, with no restrictions placed on us by work and children. Cruise ships full of grey-haired happy people beckon; that golf membership we never had the time for can now be ours. It is the common expectation of most people that retirement from work will usher in some sort of golden age where all our wishes come true.

It is simply not true. We have believed a lie.

So many retirees are not happy at all. Statistically, the divorce rate spikes in the years immediately following retirement, as spouses who previously spent much time apart are suddenly forced together. Many struggle with the unstructured time they now have to fill. Men, in particular, often struggle with feeling that they are not being useful or contributing to society. Depression rates increase as people struggle with accepting that the unrealistic fairy tale of retirement they expected is not what the reality turned out to be.

I love to play golf when I can and often meet retirees while playing. Many have told me that they started playing golf for something to do, being unable to think of other ways to fill their time. Some play golf every day or several times a week for lack of a better option.

Men's sheds are a growing phenomenon in Australia. These are community organisations that gather men together to work on projects and socialise and are heavily supported by retirees. A co-ordinator of one of these men's sheds gave an interview recently on the radio explaining how his organisation helped retired men; he said that instead of staying at home making their wives miserable, they could come to the men's shed and be miserable there!

There is a growing realisation among the broader society that a retirement made up of a few decades of leisure is destructive mentally and physically.[1] Many others have written offering ideas and suggestions concerning hobbies and distractions we can take part in during our retirement years.[2] Most books written on the topic of retirement don't deal with problems retirees face; they simply assume retirement is the wonderful nirvana we have been promised and give us tips on how to make enough money to enjoy it when the time comes.

This book is an attempt to do something altogether more important. My aim is to help Christians think about what it means to live a life serving Jesus in retirement. The truth is that too many Christians simply conform their thinking to our broader culture when it comes to retirement; the lives of retired Christians too often look identical to the lives of retired people who don't know Jesus. Surely those who know the wonder of being saved by Jesus should have a different dream for the latter stages of our lives than to live a life of selfish indulgence!

Christians are called to be distinctive in the society we live in, like a city on a hill or a light on a stand that illuminates the whole house.[3] That cannot only apply to younger believers but also those living through their retirement years counter-culturally. We are called to take up our cross and follow Jesus,[4] to understand that serving Jesus means suffering and active service. Again, surely that applies to how we live in older age, not only to our priorities and lifestyle when younger. In all things, we need to examine our thinking and priorities to ensure they are not simply conformed to how everyone else in our society thinks.[5] We need to have our minds renewed to understand the will of God so that we can live to serve him with all our hearts, minds, souls and strength.

When Christians strive only for the self-centred leisure of the promised retirement ideal, it is not only those retirees who suffer. The local church suffers too. Many churches lack older people who are active in service and leadership. Too many mature church members spend a massive percentage of their money and time on travel, which leads to local churches not being built up by the gifts Jesus has given to them and leaving a vacuum of Christian maturity needed by their younger members. As the population of Western countries is generally ageing, this problem is accelerating.

The situation is not all negative, of course! I have had the privilege of serving side by side in my local church with many who are older than me, including a number who are retired. I know the great blessing that older believers can have in the church in terms of maturity, encouragement, prayer and service. Not all of the more senior saints have absorbed the thinking of the broader culture on the issue of retirement!

It isn't easy to come to a topic like retirement with fresh eyes as a Christian. We have a lot of assumptions and expectations already in our minds. Our challenge together in this book is to consider what serving Jesus might look like in the latter stages of life, with the time and resources we have. To do this, we need to look at what the Bible has to say on the topic. No chapter or book in the Bible deals with retirement directly; it would be helpful if Paul added some kind of appendix dealing with this issue to the first letter to the Corinthians! The Bible does, however, have a lot to say on the issues that help us frame a godly worldview about retirement and later life in general. It will tell us how to think about issues relating to identity, purpose, the church family, and death, among other things. God, in His great kindness, has also given us direct teaching on growing older as well as furnishing us with a range of examples of older believers.

Obviously, this book aims to be useful for Christians who are retired from work. Ideally, though, we should think about these issues prior to retiring. Too often, we don't think about retirement except to plan for future finances. Christians need to prepare for their service in the church and society when they have the time retirement will give them. This is a book for adults of all ages.

How might we better understand our often incorrect assumptions about retirement and consider a more godly perspective on these things? The main answer has to be by considering what the Bible has to say on this topic. We will be considering a range of books and passages from the Bible, but one of the most prominent will be the book of Ecclesiastes. This often-neglected Old Testament wisdom book was written from the perspective of an older man who looked back on his life and considered what was meaningful and what was not. His instruction will help us understand the issues around finding meaning, satisfaction and putting death in perspective.

In today's world, retirement is simply a part of most cultures and we should seek to understand how it came to be that way. As we work through these issues together, we will touch on some history and secular research on our way to looking at key Bible passages.

Section 1
Retirement is not the paradise we are looking for

Chapter 1
A history lesson:
how did we get here?

Most of us hope that we will stop working while still healthy and then spend a few decades doing whatever we want. Many expect that not only should they be able to retire as soon as possible, but the government should provide some sort of pension to support it. If a politician wants to become unpopular, all they need to do is suggest that retirement benefits be reduced or limited in some way. In France, a suggestion for a moderate change to the retirement system resulted in large crowds rioting in the streets and burning cars.[1] The Italian government also faced civil unrest after suggesting a higher retirement age due to a national financial crisis.[2] After all, most reason, how dare the government reduce my pension that I deserve? I have worked hard all my life, paid my taxes, and expect to be able to enjoy my retirement in comfort. As early as possible, ideally.

Few people, however, realise that this is a quite new expectation in world history. Retirement in the form we have today was simply unheard of as recently as one hundred and fifty years ago.

In ancient times, people tended to work their entire lives, perhaps reducing their duties as they became older and less physically able. This was necessary as pre-industrial cultures were very work-intensive. Farming requires that all available people to be involved constantly; the luxury of extended leisure in your later years could not be afforded.

Retirement is not a Biblical concept. Perhaps that surprises you. The Bible was written over a very long time period and to a wide range of background cultures, but no passage describes or encourages a significant period of leisure in the latter part of life. The closest that we can find is an instruction to the Levitical priests who, while expected to retire from active service at age fifty, were instead to transition to help the younger priests instead of sitting back and being waited on.[3]

In most traditional cultures in ancient times and today, older people played a most significant role in society. They were consulted for their wisdom and life experience. Elderly relatives who could no longer live independently lived with their children or grandchildren, participating in home life as they were able to. We see something of this function for the older members of a Christian family in Paul's instructions for older men and women to train and mentor younger Christians.[4]

The modern concept of retirement has its origins in the actions of Chancellor Otto von Bismarck in 1883.[5] Facing political pressure, Bismarck agreed to pay a pension to any nonworking German over the age of 70. This was significantly higher than the life expectancy of the time, which was around 40. Bismarck made this concession knowing it would not cost him much, as very few people lived to that kind of age in 1883! In 1916, the German parliament reduced this age to 65.[6] This decision introduced the principle that the government should fund a retirement pension. It also introduced the magic number 65 as the age that people can officially retire.[7] Despite massive changes in life expectancy and culture and the economy, even today 65 is considered to be the average age that you can officially expect to retire from regular work.

The concept of retirement was promoted for different reasons in the United States of America in the 1930s.

The Great Depression created extremely high unemployment rates, a situation made worse because older workers were not retiring to make way for younger workers. Governments attempted to make retirement attractive to older workers, but very few people were interested in it and preferred to keep on working. President Franklin D. Roosevelt introduced the Social Security Act of 1935 to ease the passage of workers into retirement; it was a plan for workers to contribute to their own insurance, paid out to retirees. This was the forerunner of modern superannuation plans which are now foundational to retirement planning.

Despite the great need for older workers to retire, the idea of extended leisure in ones' older years did not become attractive quickly. Even as recently as 1951, there were roundtable discussions about how to encourage retirement among Americans.[8] It was not socially acceptable to stop working only to engage in leisure, at least among the middle classes.

Over the following decades, the concept of retirement moved from a fringe idea to become the accepted common expectation that it is today. Engaging in leisure for the last few decades of your life became something to aspire to, save for, and expect. This was fuelled by the financial services industry that helped people save for their retirement and was bolstered by the many industries that have identified retirees as a growing market with money to spend. Luxury travel has become a significant growth industry due to the prevalence of older people with substantial financial resources.

Most people living in the Western world now see

retirement as a fundamental right. It is expected. The culture has moved from it being unthought of, to being unwanted, to being expected. As we will see in coming chapters, this might seem like progress, but it has led to a range of unintended adverse effects on society, relationships, and mental health. It is destructive for people to fail to be engaged in something productive; on that point, the Bible and modern social science agree.

The expectation of retirement places massive financial pressures on world governments. The largest age demographic in Western countries, the so-called 'Baby Boomers' born in the aftermath of World War 2, are currently retiring in large numbers. Fewer workers are supporting an ever-increasing number of retirees, who are funded both by governments and their own savings. Most countries have responded to this financial burden by raising the retirement age, albeit slowly, to reduce backlash from a population that is highly resistant to threats to their expected rights. Retirement pensions are also being reduced in generosity with financial incentives given for people to save for their own retirement, rather than being supported by the taxpayer. This expectation of a fully funded retirement is unsustainable, but no politically acceptable solution is obvious.

This quick review of history should, at the very least, make us question our assumptions about retirement. We might think we have a right to a few decades of doing whatever we want later in life, however this is a new idea historically. It is proving to have severe consequences for society, our mental health, and the church.

Just because an idea is widely accepted doesn't mean

it is correct or helpful. There was a long time in history when everyone believed that the sun revolved around the earth. In relatively recent times, it was widely believed that some races were genuinely inferior to other races.[9] Almost no-one holds to either of those ideas anymore, for the evidence against them is too strong, and the social consequences of holding to those ideas are too terrible. Perhaps in the future, we will look back at our view of retirement in the early 21st century with horror as we better understand the impact this view has on our economy and the church.

As Christians, if we are aiming for a Biblical worldview in all things, it is not enough to absorb what the current culture says about a topic and then search for some kind of proof text to back it up. It is not enough to think that unless the Bible says something directly about the issue, we can go ahead and think about it like those who don't know God. It is true that the Bible says nothing about the age of 65 being a suitable time to stop working, and it does not address the idea of retirement in the modern sense. That doesn't mean that God is silent on the issue. God has revealed a great deal to us in the Bible about identity, purpose in life, and where our hope lies. As we understand these fundamental building blocks of a Biblical way to see the world, our view on retirement needs to change.

Chapter 2
What makes your life worthwhile?

When people retire after a lifetime of work, they commonly expect that they will feel wonderfully free and fulfilled because they can finally do whatever they want to do. It doesn't tend to work out that way. After a honeymoon period of sleep-ins and the long-awaited holiday, it is more common for retirees to struggle with feelings of depression. The adjustment from paid work to leisure is difficult psychologically.[1]

One reason for this is that the way we think about ourselves, our worth and dignity, is so easily tied up in what we do. When we can no longer be identified by the work that we do, and we feel that we are not contributing productively to society, we often feel we are worth less than we were previously.

To help us understand the concepts of identity and worth, we're going to look at three culturally acceptable places that we often look to in order to feel valuable. We will also seek the Biblical answer to what makes us valuable which will help us understand why retirement can be so unhelpful for us. It will also help us think about work and ageing more positively.

1. We often measure our worth by what we do

When you meet someone new for the first time, what topics tend to come up in the first few minutes? Once you've exchanged names, it is so easy to move to asking, "So what do you do?" Without intending to be judgemental, we then make assumptions about the person we have just met based on their answer to that question. If they are a doctor, then we assume they must be clever and wealthy. If they are an accountant, we might conclude that they have a steady job, albeit not a particularly exciting one! If they are unemployed or work in some unskilled job, we often struggle to know what to say next. Whatever their answer, it is easy to subconsciously rank ourselves against this new person. Our work is one of the key things that gives us status in our society.

Work is essential for us. We were made to be workers.[2] Although so many people speak of work as a necessary evil, the Bible describes work as a positive thing. After all, God is described as a worker,[3] and it makes sense for us to work as our Father does. We are given the task of work looking after God's world.[4] The Bible describes people working in all kinds of different industries due either to their skills and interests[5] or the necessities of life.[6] The idea of a "working class" who are inferior in some way to those whose wealth enables them not to work is an idea that springs from societies that had huge social class divisions; workers are never seen as inferior in the Bible.

When the Old Testament law spoke of work and rest, God put the balance at six days of work and one day of rest. While the discussion of whether the Sabbath applies or not today is not the subject of this book, note the ratio. Six to one. God expected that his people would work far more than they rested. That was the intended balance of things. We are made to work and be productive more than we are to rest, and work is never described as a negative thing anywhere in the law of Moses.

The Bible teaches rather that there is something wonderful about a hard day's work. As the Teacher of Ecclesiastes wrote so many years ago:

> *Behold, what I have seen to be good and fitting is to eat and drink and find enjoyment in all the toil*

with which one toils under the sun the few days of his life that God has given him, for this is his lot.[7]

(Ecclesiastes 5:18)

We inherently understand this concept. Completing a task brings us satisfaction. Reaching a milestone at work, and feeling that our labour has been worthwhile, brings us joy. Whether we are an accountant who has successfully balanced the books, a bricklayer who can see the wall he carefully constructed, or a surgeon who see the practical results from his operation in a better life for his patient, productive work is a good thing.

By the time of the Protestant Reformation, some of this Biblical emphasis on the nobility of work had been lost. A class structure was well entrenched, with peasant farmers generally understood as less significant than those of greater social standing. Despite this, the Reformers emphasised that all work was noble when done to the glory of God. The washerwoman could glorify God through her work just as well as the prince.[8]

We still recognise the value of work, and we tend to rank people based on their work and contribution to society. Those who are unable to work due to unemployment or disability generally find the experience incredibly frustrating; we know, deep down, that work is a good and noble thing that we should aspire to. Those who do not have any useful work to occupy them can easily end up living in destructive ways. Youth boredom and unemployment have a direct correlation to crime rates; the rich kids of Instagram waste many thousands on expensive toys in an attempt to find some meaning in their idle lives.

Work is good, but not the main place to find our identity

There is something good about enjoying our work and finding some satisfaction in it. Like all good things, however, it is so easy to twist it into something less honouring to God. Work is indeed a noble thing to be engaged in to the glory of God, but we often work only for our own glory and reputation and reward. We find our work is what defines us and where we can measure the success or failure of our lives. Instead of a component of our service to God, it can easily take a more significant role in our identity.

Having meaningful work is a good gift from God. Like all good gifts, we can end up worshipping the gift and not the Giver.[9] With work, this can mean that we start to find our value mainly in what we do. We stop thanking God for the skills and opportunities we have had that enable us to work, and we start to think that we deserve our reputation and achievements.

A more complete Biblical understanding of work has to take into account that our work is made more difficult by sin. Adam originally had meaningful, productive work to do in the Garden; after the fall, his work was made difficult by the presence of thorns and thistles. It is work bent out of its original design by the curse that we experience today. We still have glimpses of the satisfaction that comes from work, but we also feel the futility and frustration of work. Whatever we do, it will become repetitive. Even neurosurgeons do variations on the same operations day by day! However much we accomplish, it never brings lasting satisfaction or enjoyment.[10] We start to feel like we are in an endless loop that we cannot wait to get out of, and retirement looks like the perfect solution to the frustrations of work.

The problem is that retirement doesn't end up making us feel better. We might be rid of the frustrations of work to some degree, but we also miss the purpose and satisfaction and status that work provides us. We were made to work, and we can no longer define ourselves by our careers. That empty feeling that many retirees experience could well be related to the fact that we were made to work, as our Father works, and not to simply spend time in leisure.

There is another related place that we look for meaning as well:

2. We often measure our worth by what we contribute and achieve

It is normal for us to want our lives to mean something. We would like to make a difference to the world, to leave the world better than how we found it. Simply making money doesn't satisfy many people; we search for something more than that.

Despite the difficulties that come with work, paid employment is where most of us find satisfaction and a sense of purpose.[11] Being in the same workplace as others gives the sense of many working together towards the one goal. Reflecting on a finished project or a satisfied customer brings us pride and joy.

Our contribution to our workplace or society is often recognised by others as well. If we have served in a workplace well, this will likely be recognised by others, and we may get a raise or be promoted. Perhaps significant achievements will even be recognised with some kind of award or ceremony. Even if we don't look for such accolades, others may notice the impact we have on our workplace or the wider society.

The most obvious way we measure our worth is by our salary and standard of living. If we contribute to our company well, we should be reimbursed well. It is human nature to measure our success by our income and all that comes with that: houses, cars and holidays. This gives us a point of comparison to other people.

It is when we reach middle age that we can often start to realise that our achievements are limited and that there is much that we won't be able to accomplish in this life. We may have achieved a great deal in our chosen field, but the further we go through life, the fewer alternative options are available to us. We might never get to travel the world. We may never achieve everything we wanted to achieve. That realisation hits home for many people, and they buy that sports car and get a face-lift in the hope of looking and feeling younger, like they have the hope of doing everything they want to in this life. But however capable we might be, we will never achieve everything we want. We cannot do it all. We can do some things well, accomplish a limited number of things, and make a difference to society in some minor ways. But we cannot do all we want to do.

On top of this, all of us are replaceable. None of us is capable of remaining in our positions forever. Even if you are a CEO or a business owner or some other key person in an organisation, the company will continue on if you retire. In time, another person will fulfil your role. We like to flatter ourselves that no-one can do what we do, but it is not true in the end. Whatever we achieve, however important we are, one day we will be replaced.

Contribution and achievement are good but they are not the main places in which to find our identity

If we base our self-worth on what we have contributed to society and what we have achieved financially, the transition to retirement will be very difficult. When we no longer work, our most valued means of contributing to society and achieving new things is removed from our lives.

Many retirees start to question their own worth after a period spent indulging only in entertainment and chasing their pastimes. Watching large amounts of television or reading large quantities of books might pass the time, but these things don't contribute much to the wider world. The lives of retirees can easily become self-indulgent rather than productive.

Of course, it is possible to live in a way that continues to contribute to society in retirement, as many do. There are a great many retired people who volunteer in society in valuable ways in schools, community outreach, aged care facilities, and in churches. All of us need to feel needed. We need a reason to get up in the mornings. But even if you remain active and other-person-focussed in retirement, if you start to slow down and become less capable than you once were, using this as a basis for your identity will become an issue for you again. Any identity that is based only on what you can achieve or contribute, whether paid or unpaid, will break down once we cannot do what we once did.

3. We often measure our worth by how society judges us

While the work we do or the achievements we have reached might be measurable, understanding our self-worth is more subjective. How we feel about ourselves is not something we can quantify on a graph. A lot of our self-worth tends to come from knowing how others think about us.

This does change significantly depending on the wider culture that you live in. For example, Western cultures value authenticity and self-expression, so living in a way that makes you happy will be admired and respected. Eastern cultures will not see the value in authentically living a life that doesn't lead to wealth and measurable success, so it is possible to be highly respected in one culture and dismissed as being of low value by another culture.

In addition, the people you closely associate with might have their own, often unwritten, criteria for assessing worth. If your close friends are all successful businesspeople, they might value the suits you wear and the way you present yourself very highly. In contrast, if your close friends are all surfers, formal dress might be completely irrelevant, and your ability to ride big waves and the brand of surfboard you own might matter far more.

If you hold a senior position in a company or a respected role in a church, you might find that others start to ask for your opinion on things. They assume that your role and experience mean that you will be someone whose opinion matters. Without consciously realising it, enough of these interactions starts to make you feel like you are someone important. The same is true of anyone with enough experience in a field, from sports through to raising children. You can start to see your role as the fount of knowledge to others, and your worth is in the experience you have.

Your age also has a significant impact on where you think you fit in the world. If you are in a Western culture that values youth and beauty, just being in the young adult age bracket makes you important. Music and movies tend to be marketed at younger people. Older people spend a great deal of money and time attempting to look younger than they really are. Employers tend to look to younger people to fill positions, while more mature people find it far more difficult to find employment. Those who are older can start to look back with longing on their younger years while feeling on the outside edges of society.

It is the opposite in Eastern cultures. Age and experience are valued highly. It would be natural for younger people to consistently seek out the advice of those older in their families and social circles. Older relatives are respected and often visited and intergenerational living is valued. If you live in a culture like this, age means respect, even if you haven't done anything to earn it other than remain alive for a longer time than other people.

Having the respect of others is good, but it is not the main place to find our identity

When people retire, especially in Western cultures, it is common to feel less respected and valued by others. The younger employees no longer seek out your knowledge in the workplace. Your children might be grown up with their own busy lives and they don't visit you as often as you'd like. So much of popular culture is geared to those in much younger age groups, reinforcing the feeling of being on the outside looking in.

If you find your self-worth in what others think of you or in the things your culture values, your sense of identity is on shaky ground. You might feel more or less valuable and important just based on how old you are rather than who you are or what you have done. Your sense of worth might fluctuate depending on which group of people you associate with at the time.[12] You will find yourself lacking contentment as you are constantly looking for the approval of other people or some external measure that tells you where you fit.

In Jesus: the only reliable place to find our identity

It is human nature to look for our sense of worth in where we fit in society, what we have done, or what others think of us. The big problem with this is that basing our identity on these kinds of things is unreliable. There is a better, Biblical place to find our value. If we trust in Jesus as our Lord and Saviour, we are of infinite value in the sight of God. This is where our worth truly lies.

The apostle Paul puts it this way in Philippians 4:3-11:

> *³For we are the circumcision, who worship by the Spirit of God and glory in Christ Jesus and put no confidence in the flesh- ⁴though I myself have reason for confidence in the flesh also. If anyone else thinks he has reason for confidence in the flesh, I have more: ⁵circumcised on the eighth day, of the people of Israel, of the tribe of Benjamin, a Hebrew of Hebrews; as to the law, a Pharisee; ⁶as to zeal, a persecutor of the church; as to righteousness under the law, blameless. ⁷But whatever gain I had, I counted as loss for the sake of Christ. ⁸Indeed, I count everything as loss because of the surpassing worth of knowing Christ Jesus my Lord. For his sake I have suffered the loss of all things and count them as rubbish, in order that I may gain Christ ⁹and be found in him, not having a righteousness of my own that comes from the law, but that which comes through faith in Christ, the righteousness from God that depends on faith- ¹⁰that I may know him and the power of his resurrection, and may share his sufferings, becoming like him in his death, ¹¹that by any means possible I may attain the resurrection from the dead.*
>
> (Philippians 4:3-11)

Paul had a great many reasons to find his worth in earthly things. He came from the right people and family, was educated in the proper traditions, had a solid moral code, and was respected by his peers. In the end, he describes all these things as rubbish in comparison to knowing Christ. However good these things might be, in the end, they are far inferior to being a Christian.

How can this be? We naturally place a great deal of value on what we do and what we have achieved and who we are in the eyes of others. How is trusting Jesus better than this? There are at least three reasons.

1. Jesus gives us the security we cannot find anywhere else

As we noted earlier in the chapter, basing our self-worth on our employment or how others view us is not that satisfying. Retirement puts that into sharp relief for us. Retired people can feel of lower value because they are not accomplishing what they once did.

Trusting Jesus is better than this. If we trust in Jesus, we know that we have a secure status that cannot be taken away. We are declared to be right before God because of what Jesus has done for us.[13] We can be sure that nothing can separate us from the love of God in Christ Jesus our Lord.[14] This is reinforced by the description of believers being children of God,[15] a permanent state, not one that will change.

Trusting Jesus makes us perfect in God's sight,[16] and our status before God doesn't change when we retire or grow older. Older believers who suffer frailty and disability are no less valuable in God's sight than young, strong believers who are in the prime of their lives.

2. Jesus gives us eternal value which doesn't change as we get older

Even if you have a rich and fulfilling life in every way, one day you will die. Even if you maintain the respect of others and feel a great sense of self-worth, one day it will come to an end. If the best we can hope for is a good life now, we are not aiming high enough.

One of the great benefits of coming to trust in Jesus is receiving eternal life[17] as well as freedom to live life to the full now.[18] Christians hope not just for a life that is respected and useful now but also for a life that stretches beyond our death into eternity. We hope for heaven where we can praise our good God and serve King Jesus in the power of the Holy Spirit forever.

Every other place we look for self-worth is temporary. Even the greatest of lives is barely remembered a generation or two later by those who follow. Christians have a better place to find our self-worth; we are valued children who live to worship our God and to live godly lives serving him today. This has value now as well as the life to come.[19]

3. Jesus does not save us due to our achievements or who we are

Christians are saved not because of what we have done or who we are but solely rely on Jesus for his work in saving us.[20] That is a most freeing idea if you think about it. It's not about you; it is about Jesus! We don't need to earn our way to heaven. We don't need to work hard to impress God because we are incapable of doing this. Whether you are a multi-millionaire or a disabled pensioner, you can only come to be a child of God through trusting in Jesus as your Lord and Saviour.

This puts all our focus on our work and achievements into quite a different perspective. The thing that matters most is our relationship with Jesus. All the other things we look to for our self-worth are far less important. It doesn't matter in the end whether the culture thinks you are of great value or not; what matters is what God thinks. And God bases his opinion of you on what Jesus did in your place, not on what you have accomplished.

The apostle Paul understood this. He mentions in several places that he can only boast in Jesus and not his own accomplishments.[21] Whether you have accomplished much or little in your life, it is whether you trust Jesus that matters most. You will show your trust in Jesus through what you do,[22] of course, but even these good works don't give us a basis for boasting. The good we do now is only possible by God's work in us.[23]

In the end, one of the reasons that retirement is so hard for so many is because it batters our sense of worth. If we remember that our worth is not based on our work or our contribution to society, but only based on what Jesus has done for us, that will help a great deal. You are not valuable only because of what you do; you are valuable because Christ died for you.[24]

Chapter 3
Doing nothing can kill you; the need for purpose

After a busy working life, the idea of relaxing and doing very little tends to sound like a wonderful idea. And it is, to a point. Most of us certainly need more time to rest and relax, and retirement seems to be the perfect opportunity to do just that.

But what happens after you are well-rested? A month or two months after you retire? Based on average life expectancies in the Western world, you are still likely to live for several more decades. That's a lot of time. If your only plan for those few decades is to go to restaurants, watch TV, and travel, is that enough for you? Do you think this will energise you and give you a reason to wake up in the morning?

Most of us are not that good at doing nothing. We become bored. When we don't have a purpose in life, we lose motivation for all other aspects of our lives as well. That never-ending holiday called retirement might not be as much fun as you dream it will be.

Current health advice

The danger of being idle and lacking purpose is not just a problem anecdotally; research and health advice confirms the inherent risks of long-term lack of purpose. Clinical Psychologist Derek Milne, for example, lists 'finding meaning in life' right at the top of his recipe for happiness in retirement.[1] In the absence of work as a driving factor and source of meaning, many retirees face a significant risk of mental health issues, particularly depression.

A sedentary life often leads to a rapid decline in function for retirees. As the common saying goes, "you need to use it or lose it". Those who stop work and melt into a life of passive leisure do start to lose mental abilities and general motivation. This is recognised by the health profession, with occupational therapists encouraging activity for those in aged care settings and public health messaging encouraging seniors to be active.

Like many other psychology books, Milne's solution to finding purpose in life is to make your own meaning. This could be by volunteering, taking up a hobby of some kind, or getting involved in a social group. If you don't have something that gives you a purpose, it is too easy to fall into depression and develop a severe lack of motivation to do anything at all. While there is value to this advice, we will see later on that creating your own purpose simply does not lead to the contentment and satisfaction that we are searching for.

Ancient wisdom regarding meaning

The need for meaning and a purpose in life is not something modern; this is a topic discussed at length in the ancient Biblical book of Ecclesiastes a little under three thousand years ago. The Teacher of Ecclesiastes was a wealthy man who had lived a full life. He had everything that most of us would like to have: money, power, productive work, wisdom and reputation. Yet when he looked back at all he had done, he found it meaningless.[2] It didn't bring him lasting satisfaction. He even described it as "a chasing after the wind".[3]

Today we are told that a good retirement is one that contains the finer things in life, available to any who have enough money. This is so ingrained in our thinking that most of us never stop to think if this is true. Will it be enough? Even if we never needed to worry about money, and we could design whatever lifestyle we wanted, would that actually make us happy and content?

Perhaps you are not the kind of person who thinks about these kinds of philosophical questions. But even if you don't think much about purpose and meaning, there will come a day when the issue strikes you. A time when you thought you would be happier and more satisfied than you really are, and you start to wonder why.

It is like when you finally trade in your old car and purchase a new one. That new car is so much better than the old car. It has all kinds of new functions, and it is much better to drive. It has a higher safety rating than the old one. When you first purchase it, you proudly show it to your friends, and you are constantly amazed at what it can do. Over time, that feeling fades. The satisfaction recedes. It is still a good car, but it is now just your car. You have become used to it. It no longer brings you the joy it once did. The satisfaction that comes from new things simply does not last. In a bigger sense, the satisfaction that comes with money and possessions and lifestyle always ends up like that. It is nice for a while but doesn't last. In the words of the Teacher of Ecclesiastes, it is vanity, meaningless, a chasing after the wind.

We were made for work and play

God set up a pattern for work and rest in creation: six days of work and one day of rest. This pattern matched

God's own pattern of work and rest in the creation[4] and an opportunity to remember the great work of redemption that God achieved for his people.[5] There is an important principle here we must not overlook. Rest is good when it is a rest **from** something. Holidays are often such a precious time because they give us a break from the everyday and allow us to catch our breath. We need to rest; God made us that way.

Having a holiday that stretches on for decades with no work to rest from does not give the same sense of relaxation. The initial few weeks or months of retirement often feel restful as they provide a break from the work that came before; after a while, the sense of restfulness decreases. Some retirees struggle to fill their days and find peace. A part of this is that we were made to work and be productive; sitting back in never-ending rest doesn't bring the same satisfaction.

A life of only leisure leads to other problems

Many look forward to retirement as being the time when you will finally get around to doing all those things you have been meaning to do. All the things that need fixing around the house will be done. New hobbies will be begun. Think of how productive you will be if you don't need to work!

All of us have good intentions, but when we have all the time in the world, we don't get around to doing very much. As the saying goes, "If you want something done, ask a busy person". Everyone knows that people who are not busy generally don't ever get around to doing things despite having more time. As the Teacher of Ecclesiastes puts it so tellingly:

> *Through sloth the roof sinks in, and through indolence the house leaks.*
>
> *(Ecclesiastes 10:18)*

The lifestyle of laziness that so easily accompanies a long leisurely retirement can mean that things we mean to do will not get done. Tasks, even important tasks, can be forgotten. And, without meaning to, we can become lazy and unproductive. We can become accustomed over time to the fact that inactivity is our new normal.

The apostle Paul raises another problem that can arise when we have too much time on our hands: we can become busybodies. Instead of being productive, we can get involved in other people's business. Paul connects this kind of interference and distraction with idleness and not working.[6] He commanded people who were not working and were instead being busybodies to be productive; their idleness was leading them to sin and bothering others. In fact, Paul later told the Thessalonian church that if someone did not heed the warnings in his letter (including the warning against idleness), they should have nothing to do with that person.[7] That person should be ashamed of their actions.

In another letter, Paul explained that this was a particular problem among young widows with too much time on their hands.[8] Instead of being busy with useful things, they spent their time gossiping and saying things they should not say. Their idleness was leading them to sin and also encouraging others down the same path. Just because Paul saw this issue with women doesn't mean it is not also an issue with idle men!

If we don't work at doing something productive, we will end up doing things we should not. As many of our mothers told us at one time, "Idle hands are the devil's playground".

An example of disappointment at retirement

The glossy brochures tell us that retirement should bring us joy and contentment as we live through our never-ending holiday. Many now strive to retire very early so they can experience this life of leisure sooner. What they discover quite early on is that you need to fill your time with something productive.

Markus Persson created a computer game named Minecraft, building it into one of the most popular games ever played. He sold the rights to Microsoft in 2014 for 2.5 billion US dollars. Mr Persson did what most suddenly wealthy people do: he bought a mansion in Beverly Hills and upgraded his lifestyle to include everything he ever wanted. His tweets seem to indicate that this has not led to the happiness he expected:

"The problem with getting everything is you run out of reasons to keep trying, and human interaction becomes impossible due to imbalance".

"Hanging out in Ibiza with a bunch of friends and partying with famous people, able to do whatever I want, and I've never felt more isolated".[9]

He didn't enjoy leisure as much as he hoped to. In more recent times, he has returned to programming.

So where can we find this elusive purpose?

As we saw earlier, secular psychologists know that we need purpose in our lives. Their recommendation is to find something to live for. In other words, create your own purpose in life. Find something you like doing and do that. Volunteer for a cause you care about. Work part-time in a job that brings you satisfaction. That is the same message being delivered to our children in schools: design your own purpose in life.

It sounds very modern and enlightened, but it doesn't work. Tim Keller explains why in his book *Making Sense of God*.[10] In the end, we will never find happiness and purpose by looking inside ourselves for meaning. We need to look to why we are here at all; we need to look at why God made us.

The Teacher of Ecclesiastes thought a great deal about purpose and labelled many things as meaningless, including wealth and achievements. After he had explored all the options, he reached this conclusion:

> [13]*The end of the matter; all has been heard. Fear God and keep his commandments, for this is the whole duty of man.* [14]*For God will bring every deed into judgment, with every secret thing, whether good or evil.*
>
> *(Ecclesiastes 12:13-14)*

In the end, the Teacher could not find meaning without including God in the picture. If this life is all there is, and meaning is only what you make of it, it is hard to find a point to anything. Including God in our thinking changes everything. If we know that we are created by God, and that one day we will face this same God, that sharpens the mind. Suddenly the reason we were put on this earth becomes clear. We should fear God and obey Him. This doesn't mean fear in the sense of being terrified of God; it means to respect God, to honour Him as God, and to serve and worship Him. True fulfilment won't come about with that new purchase or the never-ending holiday of retirement. True fulfilment will only come from seeing where we fit in reality as people made by God and answerable to God.

The apostle Paul expresses a similar idea in a few places, including in 1 Corinthians:

> *So, whether you eat or drink, or whatever you do, do all to the glory of God.*
>
> *(1 Corinthians 10:31)*

It doesn't matter if you have a high-powered job or if you are a retiree with time to spare; you are called to glorify God. To seek God's kingdom first in all that you do.[11] To build God's reputation among those you meet[12] and to make every effort towards godliness.[13]

The message of the gospel makes this even clearer for us. Through the death and resurrection of Jesus, those who believe have eternal life instead of certain punishment and death. Christians are like those who have been saved from drowning by a lifeguard or who have been given a heart transplant when it looked like there was no hope. If we understand how much we have been saved from, that has to give us purpose. Any life that doesn't include praising God and seeking to live as he intends hasn't understood the wonder of the gospel.

What does this mean for retirement?

If you are looking forward to several decades of doing nothing except leisure and relaxation, you are bound to be disappointed. That kind of retirement is sold to us as a wonderful way to live, but it simply does not provide the meaning we need. In all likelihood, you will lose your motivation for many things instead of finding some glorious peace and contentment. You might be led to sin in your idleness and neglect important things you could be doing.

As we're so used to the idea of a selfish and idle retirement, this encouragement to purposeful activity might seem disappointing. After all, shouldn't we have some time for ourselves in the latter part of our lives? I think this reaction reveals a great deal about our hearts. A life filled with the purpose of glorifying God is not the burden and distraction we might think. We don't need to work our way to please God; we have the privilege of living to honour God who already loves us. A life spent serving King Jesus is a life that is lived to the full,[14] a life that is lived the way that God made us to live. Living for Jesus instead of filling our idle time with whatever grabs our fancy will mean a fuller and more contented life, a life full of joy.[15]

It is likely that most people will find a sudden transition to full retirement to be unhelpful. Retirement is something that you should pray about and plan for well in advance. It is worth considering whether to reduce your hours over time or decide to continue to work a day or two a week until you cannot continue any more. Whatever you decide, remember that you are not obligated to do what most people do: stop working and just have a lengthy holiday for a few decades. Christian people have to use our time more productively for Jesus than that.

The reality is that all of us need a purpose in our lives. We don't need to come up with some kind of purpose to life because God has told us what our purpose is.

We should be living to glorify God. If God is real, and He made us and saved us in Jesus, our purpose is to live for God. We should seek ways to honour God through our productive activity. We should enjoy the gifts God has given us while also seeking to be actively serving others in the world God made. It is only when we start to live how God intends that we will be truly content.

Chapter 4
Death sharpens the mind

You have probably not had a conversation about death in the past week. It is the taboo topic in the modern world. It seems everything else that was once not spoken of in polite company is now out in the open. You can talk openly about your sexual orientation; you can mock religion and have strong opinions on politics; just don't talk about death. Unless you are at a funeral (and perhaps not even then), the topic never seems to come up.

Yet we need to talk about death. It is not a vague possibility that one day we will all die. The mortality rate for human beings is 100%. One hundred out of every one hundred people will die one day. With those statistics, you would think the topic would come up! However, most of us tend to push away any thoughts about death until we are forced to think about it.

It is in middle age that the realisation that we are not immortal starts to sink in for many people. Commonly called a mid-life crisis, at some point many suddenly understand that life is half over and they haven't achieved everything they wanted to. This can lead to a rush of seemingly odd behaviour like the purchase of the red sports car and a change in relationship status. The reality of death has a knack of focussing the mind. When death becomes a real prospect for us rather than simply a theoretical possibility, we start to assess what matters most in the time we have left.

As we get a little older again, perhaps around the time we retire, we might start to realise that we physically cannot do what we once could. We begin to slow down a little. Some of our friends and family members might struggle with serious illness and die. More of our social life revolves around hospital visits and funerals. Death becomes something we are forced to think about even if we don't want to. This can be a very useful thing as death gives us a clarity we can achieve no other way.

We only have one life

The Teacher of Ecclesiastes spent most of his time considering what brought meaning and purpose to his life. As he did this, he kept circling around to the topic of death. This wasn't just because he was a pessimistic 'glass-half-empty' kind of person; no, it is a critical ingredient in the discussion.

For example, if you value your reputation and think this brings you meaning, the Teacher has this to say:

> *There is no remembrance of former things, nor will there be any remembrance of later things yet to be among those who come after.*
>
> *(Ecclesiastes 1:11)*

Think about this: how many people can you name who were alive in the 1800s? Even avid students of history can probably only think of a few. Even the most important people in the world will be forgotten one day. Death means your reputation will also disappear; most who come after you will have no idea what you were like or what you achieved.

Death is the great leveller

The Teacher of Ecclesiastes explored the concept of wise living. Surely it makes more sense to live wisely and thoughtfully than to live foolishly? In many measures, of course, that is correct. There is a real benefit to living wisely. But the moment that you bring death into the equation, the difference between a wise life and a foolish life doesn't seem so great after all:

> *[13] Then I saw that there is more gain in wisdom than in folly, as there is more gain in light than in darkness. [14] The wise person has his eyes in his head, but the fool walks in darkness. And yet I perceived that the same event happens to all of them. [15] Then I said in my heart, "What happens to the fool will happen to me also. Why then have I been so very wise?" And I said in my heart that this also is vanity. [16] For of the wise as of the fool there is no enduring remembrance, seeing that in the days to come all will have been long forgotten. How the wise dies just like the fool! [17] So I hated life, because what is done under the sun was grievous to me, for all is vanity and a striving after wind.*
>
> *(Ecclesiastes 2:13-17)*

Whatever measure he used, the Teacher kept coming back to the same idea. Even if you have achieved a lot in your lifetime, you still have to die and not enjoy what you achieved.

In the end, whether we are rich or poor, wise or foolish, death comes for all of us. Death makes all the achievements of this life somewhat hollow and temporary, even if they seemed great at the time.

Death teaches us that material things don't mean as much as we previously thought

There is a common saying: "You cannot take it with

you". As Job put it when tragedy struck his family, "Naked I came from my mother's womb, and naked shall I return" (Job 1:21). The only thing that more money gets us when we die is a nicer coffin.

Again, the Teacher of Ecclesiastes puts this vividly and memorably. He describes a situation where a man who worked hard and achieved much faces the end of his life. When he dies, he needs to leave everything he worked for to someone else who did not toil for it (Ecclesiastes 2:21). The very thought of this is vanity and a great evil.

The more philosophical amongst us come to realise this absurdity about life at some stage: if death is truly the end of everything, so much of our lives become pointless. At best, we achieve something great, and then we have to give it away. Whatever we do, we can only enjoy it for a short time. Again, I'll let the Teacher from Ecclesiastes express this for us:

> *This also is a grievous evil: just as he came, so shall he go, and what gain is there to him who toils for the wind?*
>
> *(Ecclesiastes 5:16)*

Most of us spend time accumulating wealth, upgrading our house, and seeing our investments grow. We think at the time that these things matter a great deal because everyone seems to be working towards the same end. In the perspective of death and the limited time we have in this life, all of that activity suddenly seems less important. It is vanity. There has to be more to life than this.

Enjoying the temporary as something good

What is worth living for, then? That is what the Teacher of Ecclesiastes was trying to work out. Although he was quick to point out the foolishness of much of what we strive for, the Teacher did note a few things that brought joy and satisfaction in our limited lifespans. One of them was finding joy in everyday activities:

> *There is nothing better for a person than that he should eat and drink and find enjoyment in his toil.*
>
> (Ecclesiastes 2:24)

Sure, life is limited, but that does not mean we cannot find joy in what we do. There is little better than looking back at a day of work well done[1] or having that feeling of contentment after a beautiful meal.[2] Just because something is temporary doesn't mean it is worthless!

It is like enjoying a good book or a favourite movie. We start reading or watching knowing that at some time it has to come to an end; that doesn't mean we cannot enjoy it before that time! Life is short, and much will not endure after our death, but there is much to find satisfaction in if we will look for it during our lives.

In fact, even taking death into account, the Teacher of Ecclesiastes points out many things in this life that are worth savouring and enjoying. They include the wife of your youth,[3] the light from the sun,[4] and all the days of your life that God might give you.[5]

While so many things in life can be appreciated and bring us joy, we need to consider what matters the most in the perspective of our limited lifespans. Even if we enjoy each day we are given, death doesn't just signal the end of our lives. It signals the time we face the judgement of God.

We face more than death; we face the judgement of God

The Bible often speaks about death, but death is not seen as a full stop or an end to everything important. No, death is not our ultimate end. After we die, we face the judgement of God.[6]

For much of Ecclesiastes, the Teacher limited his perspective to life "under the sun",[7] a life assessed only by what you can experience with your senses. In that perspective, the best we can come up with is to enjoy our lives while we can until we die. That's a pretty bleak perspective on life, even if you are an optimistic person! Once you remember that life is more than just physical existence and that we are made by God and live in the world God has made, our perspective starts to shift.

God made the world we live in, and he made each of us.[8] This makes God the one we should obey and worship.[9] The great tragedy is that people are unable to do this. Even if we live the best life possible, trying to serve God with all our hearts, we will fall short.[10] This means that the deserved outcome of the judgement we face after we die is disastrous. We face punishment from God, and rightly so. The only way we can possibly be saved from this punishment is through God's actions rather than our own.[11] And, by God's incredible grace, that is what God has done. God sent Jesus to die in our place to pay for our rebellion and failure to obey. If we trust in what Jesus has done for us, we no longer need to fear the judgement of God.[12]

God looks on those who trust Jesus and sees that our debt is paid, and we are accepted as God's children.[13]

How does knowing this change what we live for in this life? Well, it changes everything! If there is a judgement day, and God is the judge, we will want to live in a way that God assesses to be good. It is no longer enough for us to enjoy food and drink and work; if we ignore God and what he has done for us in Jesus, judgement awaits us.

Jesus raised this issue with some people who questioned him about a disaster they had heard about. Pilate, the Roman governor, had brutally killed some Jewish people and even mixed their blood with the sacrifices on the altar in the temple. This was terrible government oppression that also showed no respect for Jewish religious practices. The crowd surely expected Jesus to be outraged at the government, but instead, he answered them by saying this:

> *"Do you think that these Galileans were worse sinners than all the other Galileans, because they suffered in this way? No, I tell you; but unless you repent, you will all likewise perish."*
>
> *(Luke 13:2-3)*

This was not the answer they expected. Jesus pointed out that the terrible things that happen to people are not due to their individual sin, but a terrible judgement awaits all of us. Perhaps we will be murdered by an oppressive government, or perhaps we will die after a full life at the age of one hundred; in both cases, we will face judgement from God. The proper response to seeing tragedy and death is not just to be outraged by it but to use this opportunity to assess our own lives. One day that will be us. One day you and I will die.

Look at what Jesus told his questioners to do with this idea. They needed to repent. That's not a very popular idea these days, but it is something God calls us to do on many occasions. To 'repent' literally means 'to turn', to stop going the way you are going now and turn to head in another direction. Jesus told his questioners that the reality of coming death should make them consider if they were right before God. If not, the reality of death should make them worried. They should start to realise that if they continued to head the way they were going, not trusting in Jesus, tragedy loomed over them. This thinking about death might be just what they needed to understand that they were heading the wrong way and to correct their path.

Are you right with God? If you are not a Christian, take this opportunity to think about where your life is heading. If you have a full and happy life, topped off with a lovely long retirement, is that enough? God says no. If this life is not all there is, and a judgement day is coming, investigate Jesus now. If God is real, it would be a terrible tragedy to have a great life and miss what matters most.

Living for the right things knowing God is the judge of everyone

The reality of coming death and judgement is not something only non-Christians need to be concerned with. Christians need to think about these things as well. It is easy to profess faith in Jesus and then continue to live the same way as those who don't care about God at all. That cannot be the proper response. The Christian life should have different priorities and be distinctive from the wider world.

This perspective comes through clearly in the books of 1 and 2 Kings where we read accounts of God assessing the various kings of Israel and Judah. When humans assess the rule of kings and political leaders, we look to their achievements. We care if they were popular and handled crises well; we care about their foreign policy and whether their reign led to economic prosperity for the country. Interestingly, when we see God's assessment of kings, we read almost nothing of this type. God doesn't seem to care that much if a king had military victories or was popular or led to low unemployment.[14] What God does care about is whether a king is faithful to Him or not. If a king led the people to worship the true God, he was assessed as a good king. If a king led the people to worship other gods, he was assessed as a bad king. Faithfulness to God is the measure of a good life in God's eyes.[15]

Living life like everyone else around us, prioritising the building of wealth to enjoy a hedonistic retirement, surely cannot be assessed as a faithful life by God. That kind of life might bring us honour with our family and be celebrated by our culture, but it is God who we face on Judgement Day, not our parents or our next-door neighbours. The reality of life being short and death being certain needs to change what we live for.

Well, what then should we live for? The apostle Peter helps us with this. After he has explained that the world will end and God will come in judgement, his conclusion is this:

> [11]*Since all these things are thus to be dissolved, what sort of people ought you to be in lives of holiness and godliness,* [12]*waiting for and*

hastening the coming of the day of God, because of which the heavens will be set on fire and dissolved, and the heavenly bodies will melt as they burn! ¹³*But according to his promise we are waiting for new heavens and a new earth in which righteousness dwells.* ¹⁴ *Therefore, beloved, since you are waiting for these, be diligent to be found by him without spot or blemish, and at peace.*

(2 Peter 3:11-14)

Peter says that Christians should live lives of holiness and godliness in light of the coming judgement. 'Holiness' simply means 'to be set apart' or 'to be different'. Christians should be holy people, people who live differently from the wider world. This difference can be described as 'godliness', which is a life that strives to please God. A godly life seeks to love what God loves and hate what God hates. If you strive for godliness, it will mean that you will be making every effort to live as God outlines in the Bible and to serve God well in all that you do. We will be seeking diligently to deal with problems in our lives so we might be without spot or blemish in God's sight (v14).

This diligence towards godliness is hard to reconcile with a lengthy self-indulgent retirement. At the very least, we need to keep working on our holiness, to work at being different to everyone else for the sake of Jesus. We need to live for God and not simply to please ourselves.

So what's on your bucket list?

You may have heard of the concept of the 'bucket list.' This is a list of activities you hope to achieve before you 'kick the bucket' (a colloquial term for death). The idea of a bucket list is a very recent concept, with no usage of the phrase before 2004,[16] but it is undoubtedly in everyday use now. Common bucket list items include adventurous activities like climbing a mountain or cultural experiences like visiting the Louvre in Paris. It is a term that captures the thinking around the modern view of retirement so well; you need to make the most of the time you have to do all the things that are important to you. A 'bucket list' is simply a way of codifying self-indulgence.

John Piper described something of this in his famous illustration:

"I will tell you what a tragedy is. I will show you how to waste your life. Consider a story from the February 1998 edition of Reader's Digest, which tells about a couple who "took early retirement from their jobs in the Northeast five years ago when he was 59 and she was 51. Now they live in Punta Gorda, Florida, where they cruise on their 30 foot trawler, play softball and collect shells."

At first, when I read it I thought it might be a joke. A spoof on the American Dream. But it wasn't. Tragically, this was the dream: Come to the end of your life—your one and only precious, God-given life—and let the last great work of your life, before you give an account to your Creator, be this: playing softball and collecting shells.

Picture them before Christ at the great day of judgment: 'Look, Lord. See my shells.' That is a tragedy. And people today are spending billions of dollars to persuade you to embrace that tragic dream. Over against that, I put my protest: Don't buy it. Don't waste your life."[17]

In the perspective of coming judgement from a real God, all of our bucket list items start to look quite foolish. Maybe softball and shells are not your thing, but all of us are guilty of placing emphasis in the wrong places. A retirement spent playing as much golf as you can or reading the one hundred books you should read before you die seems kind of shallow. At the time, the activities might bring us some happiness; in eternity, these things have little value.

Some years ago, I sat down for coffee with a traveller from Canada. He had quit his job and left all he knew to head to the other side of the world and surf. By the time I met him, he had been surfing his way around Australia for several months already. When I asked him what his plans were, he took a list out of his pocket. He told me that he intended to work his way through this list of great experiences. What he had never thought about was why he was doing this. I asked him whether completing that list would make him happy. It was something he had never considered. In the end, he realised that he was running away from problems at home, and he was trying to find purpose and fulfilment in a self-indulgent life. This man came to know Jesus as his Lord and Saviour some weeks after this. Once his perspective on life changed, and he came to know his Creator and Judge, he changed his life. He headed back to Canada, faced the problems he had run from, and sought to live a life more about God and less about himself.

Learning at a funeral

I know you probably don't like to think about death, but you should. You learn more at a funeral than you ever could at a party.[18] Life is short, but filling it with self-indulgence won't bring you the happiness you hope it will. The truth is that God made you, and one day God will judge you. Filling your life with accumulated wealth and bucket list experiences won't excuse you from death and judgement. A good and full life has to have God in the centre of it.

We will explore some possibilities for serving God well later in life in a few chapters' time, but for now, I want to leave this concept ringing in your ears. God is the one who assesses your life, not you, your parents, or your neighbours.

When you face God on the Last Day, don't come with your bucket list. Don't come with an impressive portfolio of possessions and achievements. Come as one who understands that Jesus is the only way to be right on the Day of Judgement, and come as one who has strived for holiness and godliness diligently even in retirement.

Chapter 5
Don't substitute 'retirement' for 'heaven'

Towards the end of your working life, you might find yourself looking out the window, dreaming of what the future might look like. On those slow Tuesday afternoons, or on those days when work seems so difficult or soul-crushing, you need to know that something better is coming.

What is it that you dream of when you think of the future? The easy and immediate answer for many in their 50s and 60s is 'retirement'. We look forward to retirement as the time when we will no longer have to work. We will be able to do whatever we want to do. In our idle moments, we might build up retirement as the answer to all of our current problems. It is the cultural hope for the future, the carrot that drives us forward, and the pot of gold at the end of the rainbow. Retirement offers freedom from the work we often do not enjoy and the opportunity to spend time in activities that we get to choose.

We need something to hope in. When we think of the future, we need to know that it will be worth living for. We need to know that there is something to look forward to. The problem is that retirement will not solve our problems. If what we live for is the long holiday after our working life, we are not thinking big enough.

A better hope: heaven

The ultimate future hope for Christians is not retirement, but a life spent with God forever. We mustn't substitute 'retirement' for 'heaven'; that is exchanging something good for something perfect. The Christian hope is so much bigger than a rest from work in the latter part of our lives.

Those who trust in the God of the Bible and what he has done for them have always looked forward to a life after death. King David, who lived roughly three thousand years ago, looked forward to a life with God after he died. In his famous Psalm 23, after recounting the wonder of being one of God's people through good and bad times in this life, David wrote:

> *Surely goodness and mercy shall follow me all the days of my life, and I shall dwell in the house of the LORD forever.*
>
> *(Psalm 23:6)*

David looked forward to dwelling with God not just in this life, but "forever".[1] When David's child died as a result of his sin with Bathsheba, David understood that his son could not come back to him. Despite this, there was still a future hope in David's mind. He looked forward to the day he would be reunited with his son after death.[2]

Admittedly, the concept of heaven as eternal life with God was pretty shadowy in the time of David. We can read of the confidence that the ancient believers had in the future due to their God,[3] but they didn't have a clear idea of what this might involve. As God's work among his people continued over time, we are told far more about what this future hope would be like.

The prophet Isaiah ministered through a most difficult time in Israel's history: the fall of the southern kingdom and the exile into Babylon. In the midst of those dark times, one of the major themes that come up in the last few chapters of Isaiah is the eternal future hope that God's people have to look forward to. Even during times of weeping now, believers can look forward to this:

17"For behold, I create new heavens and a new earth, and the former things shall not be remembered or come into mind. 18But be glad and rejoice forever in that which I create; for behold, I create Jerusalem to be a joy, and her people to be a gladness. 19I will rejoice in Jerusalem and be glad in my people; no more shall be heard in it the sound of weeping and the cry of distress. 20No more shall there be in it an infant who lives but a few days, or an old man who does not fill out his days, for the young man shall die a hundred years old, and the sinner a hundred years old shall be accursed. 21They shall build houses and inhabit them; they shall plant vineyards and eat their fruit. 22They shall not build and another inhabit; they shall not plant and another eat; for like the days of a tree shall the days of my people be, and my chosen shall long enjoy the work of their hands. 23They shall not labor in vain or bear children for calamity, for they shall be the offspring of the blessed of the LORD, and their descendants with them. 24Before they call I will answer; while they are yet speaking I will hear. 25The wolf and the lamb shall graze together; the lion shall eat straw like the ox, and dust shall be the serpent's food. They shall not hurt or destroy in all my holy mountain," says the LORD.

(Isaiah 65:17-25)

Isaiah knew that the people he was writing to were struggling. The message he delivered from God was one of hope in a world that would be so much better than their current experience could imagine.

The future hope for believers meant the end of so much

that was evil and difficult in the current world. There would be no more weeping (v19) and no more people who die prematurely (v20). This future would involve settling in their own houses and enjoying the fruit that comes with peace (v21), something quite different from a life in exile away from home. They would have work that brings enjoyment and satisfaction (v22). There would no longer be conflict in the animal kingdom, for the curse on the world due to sin will be removed (v25).

Now, I do pray that all of this is encouraging for you as well, but it's not even the best bit! God's people were suffering under the just judgement of God during the time Isaiah wrote chapter 65. Into that context, Isaiah promises that the future will see a restored relationship with God. In fact, God will care for his people to the extent that he will answer them even before they call to him (v24). This wonderful future will be due to God's work and not theirs (v17), and God will rejoice and be glad in his people (v19). The core reason that this eternal future would be so good was that God would be with them and their sin and its effects would be dealt with in full.

We who live after the time of Jesus know more than Isaiah knew about how God did this. At just the right time, God sent Jesus to earth. Jesus lived a perfect life, fulfilling the law in our place. He died on a cross, paying for the sins of all who trust in him. And he rose again, showing that our sins had been paid for. This is the good news that Christians hold dear. We believe that we are forgiven people, those who had been lost and now are found. Christians are people who know that we faced certain eternal judgement from God. Because of what Jesus did in our place, we look forward to eternal joy with God instead. What Jesus has done for us means we look forward to an eternity in heaven with God who loves us.

The apostle John explained what this would be like in his vision in Revelation 21 and 22. He described the joy of believers being united with our God as being like a bride being presented to her husband on her wedding day (Rev 21:1-2). And then we are told what this eternal life would be like:

> ³*And I heard a loud voice from the throne saying, "Behold, the dwelling place of God is with man. He will dwell with them, and they will be his people, and God himself will be with them as their God. ⁴He will wipe away every tear from their eyes, and death shall be no more, neither shall there be mourning, nor crying, nor pain anymore, for the former things have passed away."*
>
> *(Revelation 21:3-4)*

This sounds like Isaiah 65, and I am sure that that is not a coincidence. All Christians can look forward to this glorious future where all the effects of sin are gone. There will be no crying, no death, no pain; all of these are due to our rebellion against God. As Jesus has paid for all of the sins of believers in full, we will no longer suffer the effects of sin like we do in this life. We will not get sick in heaven. We will not grieve, for there will be no death. We will not be dissatisfied or frustrated, for the sin that causes all these things will be no more.

However, just like in Isaiah 65, the apostle John makes it clear that eternal life is not just about the benefits we will experience with no sin. Rather, the focus is on the relationship we will have with God. God will live with us. We will have no need to be separated from God due to our sin, and we will call God our Father. Even though Christians have a real relationship with God now because of Jesus, we will experience something better and closer than we can imagine in eternity. That is the joy of heaven: it is where our good God is. That is why Christians long to be there.

We must understand this point. Sometimes heaven is described to us as a place where we can do whatever we want to do. If you like golf, it is a never-ending game of golf where you always play well. If you like parties, it will be like an endless party with the best atmosphere. The Bible doesn't describe heaven like that at all. Heaven is not about us and our self-indulgence. The eternal hope for Christians is not that we can fulfil all our selfish dreams! Our hope is that we can spend eternity praising the God who made us, who loves us, and who saved us. Heaven is God-centred; it is all about serving God and not about serving ourselves.

Compare the pair

Why are we talking for so long about heaven in a book about retirement? It is because our modern culture too often substitutes 'retirement' for 'heaven'. Even Christians start to think this way. It is easy to have retirement as the time we dream of and long for, while heaven is something we fail to desire or even think about. How is heaven superior to retirement? Let me give you three reasons.

Firstly, heaven is eternal, while retirement is temporary. Even the best retirement will last only a few decades. Those with enough money and the health to enjoy it might have extended holidays and experience the finer things in life. But as we saw in the previous chapter, the realities of ageing and death will come for all of us. Heaven is so much better. The Christian hope is one of spending time with God forever. Dreaming of a few good years of leisure is a poor substitute for an eternity spent in a perfect world with a loving Father.

Secondly, heaven is perfect, while retirement can only at best be very good. Some people will live a retirement that does look somewhat like the glossy superannuation brochures promise. They will go on cruises and drink fine wine and stroll on the beach with their loved ones. And yes, that does appeal to many of us; it would indeed be very good. Very good, however, is not good enough. Even the most harmonious marriages include arguments; even the healthiest person suffers illness and gets old. The best retirements will include pain, mourning over lost loved ones, family conflicts, frustration and discontentment. Heaven is so much better. The eternal life Christians look forward to is one with no sin, one in which the effects of sin will be no more. We will experience life as it was meant to be. There will be no relationship problems and pain and mourning; we will experience life to the full without the bits that bring us pain and suffering.

Thirdly, heaven is God-focused, while retirement so easily becomes a selfish goal. Retirement grabs our imagination because we are self-absorbed people. It is easy for us to get excited about an extended time doing whatever we desire! While that sounds attractive, it is destructive for us in the end. God made us to be his people and to be in a relationship with him. If we spend our time focussing on ourselves, what seems so attractive will fail to satisfy us. We are made to worship God. The Christian eternal hope in heaven is where we can truly live a life that will satisfy us, for we will be doing what we were made to do: worship our good God. Living for God instead of ourselves will bring true joy. In heaven, we can do this forever without the constraints of sin that we experience now.

How can we develop a longing for heaven?

Retirement so easily looms large in our dreams of the future because we have lost the excitement about heaven that many believers in previous generations have had. There are some reasons for this.

a.   We need a more accurate understanding of how great heaven will be

When heaven is depicted in modern advertising or cartoons, there are usually clouds and harps involved. People sit around dressed in white robes. I don't know about you, but that whole image doesn't excite me much. I don't wear much white as it makes me look unwell with my pale skin and blond hair, and I have never been a big fan of harp music!

Or perhaps you think of heaven as a never-ending church service. That's what naturally comes into our minds when we think of worship. However much you like your church and enjoy worship services, most of us would struggle to get excited about a life that only consisted of one long church service.

In contrast, retirement is full of things we understand. We know what holidays are like. We have experienced many of the things we look forward to in retirement, and we have a better idea of what a life full of only those things might look like. Retirement is something we can relate to in a way we struggle to relate to understanding heaven. The Bible only has metaphors to describe heaven, word pictures to try to explain to us a reality we cannot fully comprehend. It seems easier to focus on what we know instead of some eternal future we can't quite picture clearly in our minds.

Isaiah 65 and Revelation 21 do not describe heaven as being like a never-ending church service or a community of white-robed harp players. Those passages describe heaven as like life now without the impact of sin. It is a life spent with our God in a perfect way, a life that contains relationships and work and contentment. Worship in heaven is not just a church service; it is a life that is spent praising God in all that we do (like in 1 Cor 10:31).

C.S. Lewis explained the problem we have with focussing on the concrete and not dreaming of what God has promised us:

> *"It would seem that Our Lord finds our desires not too strong, but too weak. We are half-hearted creatures, fooling about with drink and sex and ambition when infinite joy is offered us, like an ignorant child who wants to go on making mud pies in a slum because he cannot imagine what is meant by the offer of a holiday at the sea. We are far too easily pleased."*[4]

If retirement seems to you like something that will fulfil all your dreams, you are not thinking big enough.

b. We need to understand that heaven is far better than the best lifestyle now

If you dream of retirement as the great hope for your future, that means you probably live in a relatively wealthy country. You probably have a job that is not just about surviving, but you have the capacity to save some money. Your government probably provides some kind of financial benefit to retirees, and you most likely live a pretty comfortable life. None of these are bad things in themselves; they are real blessings we should thank God for! However, they do mean that we can think of our future hope as kind of an extension of what our life is like now, only a little bit better.

I live in Perth, Western Australia. Perth is a comfortable, prosperous place. For many decades, we have had low unemployment. We have a very high standard of living and a stable government. Most of the population have never experienced absolute poverty or the struggles of living during wartime or through a depression. One reason people in Perth don't seem all that interested in God is because they have a good life already. They don't see the need for God. If they have a house and car and live the lifestyle they want, why would they think they need God?

Christians living in comfortable, prosperous places may not be quite as blunt as that, but we are subject to the same kind of temptations. If life is good, it is hard to imagine heaven as being so much better than what we have now. We have all that we need and much of what we want.

We place too much importance on possessions and lifestyle. Even Christians tend to equate a good life as one in which we own our own homes and live how we want. If that's what we value most, retirement is like the ultimate expression of our values. When we do that, we make the classic mistake called 'idolatry' in the Bible: we start to worship God's good gifts rather than the gracious God who gave them to us.[5]

We need to understand that life is more than food, and the body is more than clothing.[6] We need to realise that so many things matter more than a comfortable life. Man does not live on bread alone but on every word that comes from the mouth of God.[7] Living our best life is not about indulging our every desire but living for the God who saved us.

If we are going to genuinely desire heaven over retirement, we need to remind ourselves that lifestyle and comfort are less important than God. How might we do this? It can start with prayer: we should thank God for the good gifts he gives us. That will remind us that they are gifts and that they come from a Giver. The Giver should be worshipped, not the gifts. Then we might consider spending less time looking at advertising or dreaming of holidays and car upgrades; if we fill our minds and hearts with things like these, no wonder that is what we focus our time and money on!

It is accurate to say that the best things in life are free, but we often don't live like this is true. We focus too easily on the next possession or experience that will make us happy. We need to stop this. Those who know that things are temporary, but life with God is eternal, need to aim bigger than just having better toys than those we own today.

People who live in difficult times and places seem to more easily grasp the wonder that is promised in heaven. Isaiah wrote to the exiles who experienced such immense pain and promised them a bright future; John wrote to persecuted Christians, painting a picture of perfection to come. In more modern times, the songs written by the African American slaves almost always have hope of heaven as a prominent theme.[8] When you are not satisfied with your life now, you will dream of a better life than what you currently experience. If we want to have that godly hope for heaven, we need to become less comfortable and to understand that even the best lifestyle now is nothing in comparison to the glory to come.

c. We need to have our hearts captured by how great our God is

Our hearts are idol factories; we are made to worship something and live for something. This means that simply trying hard not to live for possessions and a more comfortable lifestyle is not enough in itself. Even if we are successful in resisting the urge to live like everyone else around us, we will find something else that captivates us. We will throw ourselves into some hobby like golf or craft or gardening, or fill our lives with family commitments. We are unable to be neutral. We need something to live for.

That is why we need to replace our dreaming of the ideal lifestyle with dreaming of our good God. Most Christians will naturally say that God is first in our lives, and we intend for this to be the case. Intentions are not enough. We cannot cultivate our love for God by simply saying we love God more, then spend all our time and mental energy working at more possessions and a nice retirement. That would be like someone saying that they love their wife and then never spending any time with them or putting any effort into their marriage!

The apostle Paul gives us good advice regarding this:

> *Finally, brothers, whatever is true, whatever is honorable, whatever is just, whatever is pure, whatever is lovely, whatever is commendable, if there is any excellence, if there is anything worthy of praise, think about these things.*
>
> *(Philippians 4:8)*

What do you think about? As we saw in our last point, if all we dream of is our possessions and lifestyle, then retirement naturally becomes the natural goal for us to aim at. Christians know there is something that is far more lovely and worthy of praise than these things. We trust in the true God, the one who sent his son Jesus to save us from our sins, who saved us when we could not save ourselves. We trust in the one who loves us and promises us an eternal future with him. However good your life might be now, this is undoubtedly better!

If we want to grow in our passion for heaven, we need to grow in our passion for God. After all, the great highlight of being in heaven is that we will be with the God who loves us! How do we grow in our passion for God? Paul says we should think about the things of God. This is not advice Paul came up with by himself. Moses told the people of God to speak of the things of God as you go about your everyday lives.[9] The first psalm encourages us to meditate on God's law day and night if we want a life as strong as a tree with an eternal future spent with the true God.[10] If God is first in our lives, we need to think about God, and we need to talk about God.

Eternal life, a relationship with God, is not limited to something that will happen in the future. If we trust in Jesus, we have eternal life right now.[11] If we value our relationship with God now, then we will look forward with longing to a time when that relationship will be face to face instead of in part.[12]

I know this seems kind of obvious, but in my experience, few Christians spend time reading the Bible and praying as part of their daily lives. There really is no substitute for regular time in God's word. That can be alone as part of a daily habit, with your family or housemates, with a Bible study group, or in a worship service at your local church. Ideally, it should be all of these things. There are so many things that compete for our attention and our hearts; if we don't carve out godly habits in God's word, we will surely end up living for something else entirely. If God doesn't seem so good, heaven will seem a poorer option than a comfortable and selfish retirement.

Why does it matter that we aim at heaven rather than retirement?

You might be wondering if this whole chapter is a bit redundant. Can't we have both? Why can't Christians live for a comfortable and somewhat self-focussed retirement and then simply head to heaven anyway? We are saved by grace, after all. Why does it matter that retirement captures our attention?

The bigger answer to this is that it always matters how we respond to God's grace. Yes, we are saved by God's grace; all we need to do is trust in Jesus as our Lord and Saviour, and we will be redeemed. Once we know how much we have been forgiven, we will love God with all our hearts and minds (as in Luke 7:47). If being saved makes no difference to how we live and what we live for, we have simply not understood how much has been done for us. Christians need to be distinctive in all kinds of ways because Jesus has died for us. I would argue that one of those ways is to see retirement not as an extended holiday, but as a great opportunity to serve God.

The more specific answer to why our goal being heaven matters so much is that it cannot help influence what we do with our lives now. If we know where we are heading, we will have a better idea of what to do as we head in that direction.

Our modern affluent cultures love the idea of a self-focussed retirement for some decades at the end of our lives. If this life is what we live for, and if you measure success through money and lifestyle, a retirement spent doing whatever makes you happy becomes the ultimate goal. If you are thinking bigger and heading to eternity with God, you cannot help but view this life quite differently.

Think about it like this. If you pack for a summer holiday at the beach, you pack swimwear and sun cream. If you pack for a winter holiday in the snow, you will pack thermal underwear and warm jackets and gloves. You prepare now for where you are heading. Hedging your bets and packing some warm clothes and some swimwear is not the most effective way to pack. Once you know your destination, you have a good idea of what is needed to prepare for it.

So what is needed as we prepare for eternity in heaven rather than retirement? Well, think about what we have learnt about what heaven will be like. It will be a life spent praising our good God. That means that it would be worth getting to know God through his Word now, and spending time actively praising him already. We also know that heaven includes a great multitude of God's people; it would make sense to build up God's people now, for we will be doing that in eternity. It would make no sense to spend all our time building wealth and going on never-ending holidays; that is like packing thermal underwear to go to the beach.

Again, the apostle Paul is helpful for us here. When we wrote to Timothy late in his life, with his own mortality in his mind, his advice for Timothy was this:

> *[7]Have nothing to do with irreverent, silly myths. Rather train yourself for godliness; [8]for while bodily training is of some value, godliness is of value in every way, as it holds promise for the present life and also for the life to come.*
>
> *(1 Timothy 4:7-8)*

Paul contrasts training in godliness with bodily training here. In this life, physical exercise is a useful thing. But if we are heading to eternity, godliness is a better thing to spend time and effort on. 'Godliness' is a strange word that means to be like God. That doesn't mean trying to be more powerful or to be in many places at once! It means being like God in his character: loving, gracious, just and faithful. Paul says that godliness is something we can train ourselves in. We can become more gracious towards others through prayer and practice. We can care more about justice by studying God's standards. We can become more faithful by working hard on doing all the things we promise others, whether large or small. Training in godliness has value "in every way"; it makes sense to work on these things rather than our earthly comfort if praising God is our ultimate goal.

One straightforward way to aim for heaven rather than retirement is through how we spend our money. Retirees tend to have more disposable income than most people, but how it is spent will reveal where our heart is. We are always willing to spend money on what is of greatest importance to us. If our budget in retirement is focussed only on self-gratification, I would argue that there is something wrong with what we love most. Just think of what might be done with your money that would bring eternal benefit. Retirees should be generous towards kingdom work, whether in the local church or world missions. There are opportunities to encourage others through hospitality as well.

A self-focussed retirement is not a big enough goal

The superannuation advertisements tempt us with their depictions of the everlasting holiday that we could spend our retirement enjoying. The reality is that this dream is not big enough for those who know what Jesus has done for them. If all we want is a nice life now, and we are not actively planning for our service to God and our growth in godliness, we are thinking like those who don't know what it means to be saved.

We are sinful people in a world under the curse of God, who look forward to a better life in eternity with the One who loves us. Don't be distracted by the shiny things that retirement offers; dream bigger than that.

Section 2
Regaining a firm foundation:
What the Bible says about age and maturity

Chapter 6
Direct Biblical teaching on age and maturity

Our view of old age most naturally comes from the culture that we have grown up in. Those who have grown up in Eastern cultures are taught to respect the elderly and listen to the wisdom of those who are older. Many who have grown up in Asia or Africa are used to the idea of grandparents living in the same household as young children. If you have grown up in a Western culture, you are far more likely to be uncomfortable with the idea of growing old. Grandparents are often living apart in retirement villages or nursing homes. The relationship between generations is nowhere near as close.

No culture perfectly lines up with the view of old age that God presents to us in the Bible. As tempted as we might be to say that our culture's understanding of age is correct, we need to slow down and listen to God's word carefully. God says a lot about age and ageing in the pages of the Bible. We will see direct teaching about growing older as well as a wealth of examples of older people living in God's world. In this section of the book, we will look closely at what God has to say about age and maturity.

Biblical cultures: the default position is respect for the elderly

The cultures of the Bible, spread across a long historical period, more closely align to traditional Eastern cultures in our world today. We notice that younger people are encouraged to respect those who are older than themselves. We see an example of this in the book of Job. Job was comforted by three friends after being devastated by his many losses. After each of his friends had spoken, a fourth man named Elihu spoke up. His speech starts with these words:

> *"I am young in years, and you are aged; therefore I was timid and afraid to declare my opinion to you. ⁷I said, 'Let days speak, and many years teach wisdom.' ⁸But it is the spirit in man, the breath of the Almighty, that makes him understand. ⁹It is not the old who are wise, nor the aged who understand what is right. ¹⁰Therefore I say, 'Listen to me; let me also declare my opinion.' ¹¹Behold, I waited for your words, I listened for your wise sayings, while you searched out what to say. ¹²I gave you my attention, and, behold, there was none among you who refuted Job or who answered his words."*
>
> (Job 32:6b-12)

Elihu was respectful to his elders, even though he burned with anger at what advice they gave to Job in his time of need.[1] This meant that he allowed them to speak first, and he listened with respect despite disagreeing. He expected wise sayings from those who were older than himself (v11). In this case, these three older friends' advice was poor, and he was prepared to disagree with them, but only once he had listened with respect. Their age meant an assumption that they would have something wise to say.

Job is a difficult book to place and date, but it is not the only place in the Bible that we see this kind of respectful stance. The elders of Israel, most naturally read as the older men who were the senior members of their families, were the ones who were called upon to make decisions and to lead.[2] The early Christian church naturally cared for widows,[3] many of whom would have been older. Paul instructed Timothy not to allow people to look down on him for his youth,[4] which shows that the assumption of the people of that time was for church leaders to be older men.

This type of respect for the elderly is something increasingly missing in our modern society. A significant proportion of older people in nursing homes do not receive any visitors. Many employers look for youth and enthusiasm over age and wisdom when selecting people to fill job vacancies. Older people are increasingly a target for criminals.

This sidelining of older people in society is a by-product of the increasing cultural priorities of youth and beauty. It is young people who grace the covers of magazines and dominate the production of music and the lead roles in movies. Sportspeople are young and strong, and actors in television dramas are young and beautiful. This emphasis leads people to long for eternal youth, searching for it in fitness, cosmetics, and increasingly in cosmetic surgery. In this kind of culture, older people cannot help but be sidelined. People feel uncomfortable being reminded that they will themselves grow older. Many aspire to youth and beauty; few aspire to old age.

The church can also be guilty of a focus on youth at the expense of the aged. Many large churches only have young and beautiful singers and musicians at the front of their services. Church music is often loud and alienating for those who are older. Many churches employ youth pastors, with only a comparatively small number employing pastors whose focus is older people in the congregation and the neighbourhood.

Older people deserve respect, and this is the default position of the Bible. It is a cultural emphasis to put the spotlight only on the young rather than a Biblical direction.

Dying at a "good old age" is a sign of the blessing of God

Long life is often described in the Bible as one of the signs of God's blessing. One of God's promises to Abraham was that he would die at a "good old age",[5] something that came about when he died at the age of 175.[6] Those who were blessed by God are often described with similar language. Gideon died at a "good old age",[7] while Jehoida is listed as dying when he "grew old and full of days".[8] Long life in the land God promised his people was also commonly listed as an outcome of following the commands God gave his people.[9]

This connection between God's blessing and long life became somewhat intuitive for the people of God. You can see this when the natural response to the crowning of a new king is the call, "Long live the king!".[10] Psalmists who pray for the blessing of a king included prayers for long life along with riches and honour.[11]

The converse is also true; God's punishment on his people often included the shortening of their lives. In the most extreme example of this, God's punishment on Eli and his sons included a curse that there would not be an old man in Eli's family line forever.[12] Not having any older people in that family was a sign God had punished them.

We can go too far with this thought; it is a general

principle rather than an absolute rule. There are many examples of godly people dying young and wicked kings living to old age. Not all older people can say they are old due to God's blessing due to their godliness. That being said, it does remain a general principle: old age is a blessing from God.

That's quite a different way of thinking about age to how our modern world views it, isn't it? Think about that next time you spot a wrinkle or realise that you have aches and pains you never used to have; it is a blessing to be given long life. Old age is a blessing from God and not a curse. That doesn't mean it is easy or glamorous, but it does change our attitude towards it. Another birthday means God has allowed our lives to continue another year. What a remarkable blessing that is, that sinful people can be sustained in such a way! Just because so many people grow old does not take away from the wonder that God blesses people with extra time in the world he has made.

The young should listen to the advice of those who are older

The book of Proverbs is full of good advice on how to live well in God's world. It is written in the voice of a father to his son,[13] but its instruction is not limited to physical families; all who read the book are called to listen to wisdom.[14] Those who listen to correction learn more even if they are already wise.[15] Whoever you are, there are always things you can learn from those who have gone before you. Those people most naturally are those of a previous generation;[16] you should grow in wisdom and experience as you grow older.

We have spent a great deal of time in this book listening to the Teacher of Ecclesiastes. While there is some debate as to the teacher's actual identity, the reason he is worth listening to is that he has experienced a great deal and reflected on what he has learned from it all. It takes many years to reach the level of experience someone like the Teacher shows in the book of Ecclesiastes. We are called to listen to his advice as someone who has lived out so many mistakes that ended up being fruitless.

In other books of the Bible, elders are described as older men who gathered at the gates of cities and were needed for important town decisions.[17] When you required wisdom, you went to the city gates to seek out the wisdom of those older than yourself. They held the authority in the town based on their age and position in the family and tribe. This is not just an Old Testament reality; Paul urges Timothy to teach that the New Testament church treat older men as fathers and older women as mothers.[18] Those who were older should be respected and listened to, with the assumption that they have something valuable to contribute.

I fear that this is something that we easily lose in the modern church. Many churches divide their communities by demographic, with older people and younger people attending different services and ministries. This removes the interaction between the generations that is assumed in places like Proverbs and 1 Timothy 5. For any sharing of life experience and wisdom, the generations need to mingle.

When I was a young adult, I was part of the planting team for a new church plant at my local university. We were predominantly passionate young Christians in our 20s. There was something special about being among friends who were in a similar stage of life to me. After a year or two, an older single lady named Wendy joined our church family. She was in her 60s; she became like everyone's grandmother. Her integration into the church family showed me that we were missing something important in not having older people. She had a natural way of caring for the others at church, inviting us to her house for a meal or to play cards. Wendy said that being in our church made her feel young; I certainly appreciated her input and different perspective on life.

If you are older and considering retirement, consider what younger people you associate with. If you only spend time with people of a similar age to yourself, you are missing an opportunity to serve others whom you can help. Whether you believe it or not, your life experience means you have something valuable to offer younger people. Look for opportunities to befriend and build up younger people in your church. Perhaps you could teach in the children's ministry. Consider inviting a young couple over for dinner. The Biblical model of the older imparting wisdom to the younger ones has great value; how can you be part of this?

Older people sometimes need the support and help of younger people

As we age, we may need help from others. We see younger people taking on such a responsibility in the Bible. One of the first practical things we read that the early church in Jerusalem was doing was providing an extensive food distribution service for local widows.[19] Not all of these widows would have been elderly, especially when the life expectancy of the time was low and many people died in the prime of life. It does seem, however, that a significant proportion of these widows were older. Once the church and its processes had been more fully established, the apostle Paul instructed Timothy to ensure that the widows being looked after by the church were over 60 and of good reputation.[20] Younger widows did not need the same help as those who were older.

Jesus himself, when he was on the cross, made sure his own mother was looked after. As the firstborn son of the family, he would usually have the responsibility to care for her in her advancing age. His impending death meant that this could not occur, but he entrusted his mother to "the disciple whom he loved" (usually interpreted as the apostle John).[21] Mary was then looked after by John in his own home; Jesus knew his mother needed help and ensured it was provided.

It is perfectly acceptable to need help as you get older. None of us wants to be in the position where we can no longer look after ourselves properly, but one day most of us will need assistance. This is an opportunity for younger generations to show love and care and for older generations to show grace and appreciation to those who minister to them.

How does this change how we think about retirement?

As we have seen, the Bible says a great deal about growing older. All of life is a gift from God, and old age is a blessing, not a curse. Ageing happens to all of us; it is a natural process, and we don't need to avoid it or hide it. Age does often correlate with wisdom; not always, but often. If we do get older, we will slow down, our health will generally worsen, and that is normal. If we are older, we should live lives worthy of respect and emulation. If we are younger, we should see the elderly with respect, listening and caring for them.

Some people are afraid of growing older. To them, retirement symbolises that they can no longer be a productive part of society. They will no longer be working full time, and they no longer have the energy they once did. The Biblical teaching is most helpful here: you are a most valuable part of society. Those who are older have a lot to offer through their life experience and wisdom. They shouldn't hide away or only associate with other older people! Younger people need the influence of older people, even if they don't always think they do. If we take the Biblical teaching about ageing seriously, we will need to design church structures to encourage mingling between generations. We will need to minister to and encourage older people who need assistance. Older people should also look for opportunities to serve others with the experience they have to offer.

Some who grow older find themselves angry and frustrated at their ill health and loss of energy. The Bible is realistic about this, far more so than the superannuation advertisements are. Your retirement is unlikely to be full of energetic activities from the time you finish work until you finally pass away. While this can be frustrating, God gives us some helpful ways to think about this slowing down in later years. We should remember that long life is a gift; even when every joint cracks and we need assistance in our day-to-day lives, God has been gracious to us. Ageing is not something unusual where we should be angry and frustrated at ourselves and everyone around us due to our limitations. We cannot reverse the ageing process. Frustration and anger don't change anything except making us harder to live with and be around! God, in His wisdom, made ageing to be part of life in this fallen world. There is no need to hide that grey hair or the fact you prefer an afternoon nap. There is still much to thank God for in our later years.

Chapter 7
The Biblical example of older believers

Stories make us understand things far better than if we were simply told facts directly. For example, I could teach a valuable lesson by saying 'you should not tell lies'. That is a true statement. Most of us would agree that it is good advice. But if we are honest, it can feel unimportant or ambiguous. If we were to teach this concept to children, we could tell them the famous story about Pinocchio, the puppet whose nose grew longer whenever he told lies. That growing nose led to his lies being discovered, so he could not deceive others as he wanted. That sticks in the mind; even if we haven't heard that story for a long time, we quickly associate telling lies with a growing nose. The basic message – that lies lead to bad consequences – is far more memorable when it is told as part of a story.

Likewise, the Bible says a lot about ageing. We see direct teaching and advice, instruction and encouragement. This is helpful and has its place. To truly understand how to live a godly life in retirement, however, we need to see real examples. And again, the Bible is full of true stories of older people. Some of them are great examples of using your age to serve God, and some of them are frankly terrible examples no one should try to follow. We will examine some of these stories in this chapter to help us see what can be done by God's people in older age.

When it comes to using Biblical characters as examples, we do need to be careful. It is very easy to wrongly apply these examples. We can fall into moralism, which is saying that this person did a good thing, so we too should do that good thing. This person did a bad thing, so we too should not do that bad thing. Life is not as simple as that. What we see in the true stories of the Bible are descriptions of real people living real lives. They are descriptions and not prescriptions. They are to be considered in context and not blindly copied by people who live in very different cultures and times. Yes, these things are indeed written for our instruction,[1] but we need to be careful not to misuse the Bible as we thoughtfully reflect on how God's older saints have lived in the past.

Positive examples of godliness in older age

Abraham and Sarah: Trusting God in older age

Abram was already an old man when God called him to leave Haran to go to the land he was promised.[2] Even though people at that time did live longer than we do today, seventy-five was not considered to be young! Abram and Sarai were wealthy people with many flocks and herds and servants and land. They had built a good life for themselves. Migration is usually the kind of thing young people are interested in doing; older people want to stay where they are comfortable and settled. Yet Abram trusted God, and it was credited to him as righteousness.[3] Instead of making excuses why it made more sense to stay where they were, this family moved a long way to a place where they did not know anyone.

Abraham[4] did believe that God would do what he promised in giving him a son when Sarai had been barren. That doesn't mean that Abraham's faith was perfect! Abraham and Sarah were impatient for God to provide them with a son, so Abraham slept with Sarai's young maidservant Hagar to produce a son rather than wait longer for the promise to come about.[5] Sarai laughed when the strange visitors told her that she would have a son within a year, for she knew that she was well past child-bearing age.[6] The son God had promised them would only be born through God performing a miracle, and their faith while they waited was less than perfect. Abraham and Sarah found it hard to wait for the impossible, yet God still gave them the promised son. The fact Isaac was born to them in such old age showed that God was completely responsible; God used older people in his plan to show that his promise came about through his strength and not theirs.

Abraham was indeed the father of many nations and used as an example of faith by Paul, the writer to the Hebrews, and James.[7] God does not limit his work to those who are young and strong! God used Abraham and Sarah despite their age and limited faith; being in your later years does not mean you cannot be of great service to God.

Moses: God uses even the elderly and unexpected in his work

God used the great prophet Moses to lead his people out of slavery in Egypt. Although we know about his secret birth and his upbringing as an adopted son of the Egyptian princess, the majority of Moses' account in the Bible took place when he was old. In many ways, Moses was an odd choice to be the greatest prophet of the Old Testament. He was an exile from his people, living in the wilderness after killing an Egyptian.[8] When God sent him to be the one to rescue his people, Moses initially refused because he was no-one special, he could not speak well, and he didn't want to go![9] On top of this,

Moses was around 80 years old when he appeared before Pharaoh, and his brother Aaron was 83.[10]

Despite all of these limitations, God used Moses in a powerful way. He led the people not only out of Egypt but through the wilderness all the way to the edge of the promised land. This was a most difficult task, dealing with multiple rebellions, mediating between God and the people, and holding the burden of leadership squarely on his shoulders. Although Moses was not permitted to enter the promised land himself, God showed it to him from the top of Mount Nebo and affirmed the covenant promises he had made to Abraham. At the time of his death, Moses was 120 years old, and his "eye was undimmed, and his vigour unabated".[11]

Moses was a reluctant leader who showed himself faithful in the most difficult of circumstances.[12] He wasn't the kind of person we might choose as a leader, someone with the energy and confidence of youth and the impressive presence and charisma that mark many modern politicians. In fact, Moses was the most humble person on the face of the earth.[13] This is yet another illustration of God's preference for using the weak over the strong in order to reveal his power.[14] Older people sometimes think that the real work of God should be left to the younger people; God did not do that with Moses. God looks to the heart, and even a humble, reluctant believer can be used in unexpected ways for God's glory.

Caleb and Joshua: Faithfulness and example even in old age

When the people of Israel first came to the border of

the promised land, God told Moses to send out 12 spies to find out what lay ahead. Each of the spies were to be a chief of their tribe, which would mean that they would be older, experienced men. When the spies returned from their task and reported that the land was both very fertile and strongly defended, the spies were divided in the advice they gave. Ten of the spies thought the land too well defended to be defeated by the untrained Israelites. Only two of the spies were confident of victory after what they saw; their names were Caleb and Joshua.[15]

Caleb and Joshua were confident of victory not because the Israelite armies were superior but because they trusted God even when they knew the hard task ahead of them. They held to their position when the majority of their esteemed colleagues disagreed. This firm trust in the power of their God to keep his promises led to blessing from God. The rest of the people suffered the penalty of dying out in the wilderness over the next 40 years, with only Caleb and Joshua remaining from that generation to enter the promised land.

These two men must have stood out among the people who crossed the Jordan near Jericho so many years afterwards. Almost all of the people were young, while Caleb and Joshua were the two old men among them. Caleb was 85 years old when he entered the promised land and had remained as strong as he was when he spied out Canaan 45 years earlier.[16] Joshua died aged 110, having seen the conquest of the promised land as God had promised Abraham so many years earlier.[17] These two men remained examples of faithfulness even in their latter years, holding leadership positions and even leading military battles as old men.

Caleb and Joshua were men who trusted God their whole lives. They knew that their God would do what he promised. Even in their latter years, they remained examples of faith and service. As Christians, we will never retire from the service of our God. We can be used to lead the younger generations. Our experience of God's faithfulness to us may inspire those who struggle with the same things we once struggled with.

Samuel: A faithful and long life

Samuel had a most unusual childhood. He was born as the result of God listening to the prayer of his mother, Hannah, who had been barren for many years. Samuel was given to God's service and spent his life serving the priest Eli at Shiloh. He was faithful to God from a very young age and also grew in favour of the people of Israel who met him when they came to worship. Samuel grew up to be a rather unusual person; he was a prophet, a priest, and a king of sorts. He spoke God's word to the people, acted as a priest before the Lord, and led the people in all kinds of ways. Samuel was the one who anointed the first king of Israel, Saul, and the greatest king of Israel, David. Samuel was unafraid to speak up against King Saul's unfaithfulness and do difficult things when required for the service of his God.[18]

Samuel was not a perfect man. Samuel appointed his sons to be judges over Israel, yet they misused their positions to take bribes and pervert justice.[19] While Samuel cannot be held to be fully responsible for his adult sons' actions, it does reflect poorly on his parenting and his wisdom in appointing them to positions they were not appropriate for.

I want us to note what Samuel said in his farewell address to the gathered people of God:

> *And Samuel said to all Israel, "Behold, I have obeyed your voice in all that you have said to me and have made a king over you. ² And now, behold, the king walks before you, and I am old and gray; and behold, my sons are with you. I have walked before you from my youth until this day. ³Here I am; testify against me before the LORD and before his anointed. Whose ox have I taken? Or whose donkey have I taken? Or whom have I defrauded? Whom have I oppressed? Or from whose hand have I taken a bribe to blind my eyes with it? Testify against me and I will restore it to you." ⁴They said, "You have not defrauded us or oppressed us or taken anything from any man's hand." ⁵And he said to them, "The LORD is witness against you, and his anointed is witness this day, that you have not found anything in my hand." And they said, "He is witness."*
>
> *(1 Samuel 12:1-5)*

These are remarkable words. After a lifetime in a public leadership position, with everyone watching him while he exercised great responsibility, he remained morally pure. Samuel did not misuse his position for his own benefit, even though he would have had the opportunity to do so. None of the people could point to any improper conduct in Samuel's life.

I pray that I would be viewed that way when I am older! Samuel would be an example for all future leaders; his leadership was peaceful and wise and respected. He remained faithful in his older age. Samuel is an example of what it looks like to follow God well all of your life.

The importance of the example of older believers cannot be overstated. Whether they realise it or not, young people need to see that a faithful life is possible. They need to know that someone can navigate the temptations of this world, the busyness of raising a family, and the challenges of leadership, and still remain faithful to God. The presence of faithful older Christians in a church is a great gift and a concrete example of the grace of God.

The apostle John: Wisdom delivered from experience

The apostle John was known as the apostle that Jesus loved.[20] He was one of the inner circle of Jesus' apostles and became a significant figure in the early church. John was a central part of the church in Jerusalem, involved in the early evangelism after Pentecost[21] and continuing his involvement at least until the spread of the gospel to Samaria[22] and the Gentiles.[23] As Acts predominantly follows Paul's ministry after chapter 9, we are not told many details about John's further ministry after this time.

John did, however, write documents that became part of the New Testament in the latter part of his life. Most commentators agree that John's gospel was written significantly later than the other three gospels. As those who followed Jesus during his time on earth were growing old, it seems likely that John wished to preserve his own eyewitness account in a way that would remain useful once he was gone. John also wrote three letters to the early church in his latter years that are preserved for us as 1, 2 and 3 John. The book of Revelation, the last book written in the New Testament, was also written by John to the persecuted church while he was on the island of Patmos.

When we read these documents produced by John, especially his letters, we can sense that these are the words of someone older. They are written by an eyewitness of Jesus. He addresses his readers as "little children"[24] and uses the term "the elder"[25] to refer to himself. The first readers would have known who was writing these letters and had immense respect for him. This is one of the inner circle of apostles! This is one of those men who went through it all with Jesus, and who had spent their lives since then spreading the gospel and building up the church! When John spoke, or when he wrote, people listened. He had something to say and made the time to write it down to make it accessible for everyone.

Of course, none of us can claim to have the experience of the apostle John! Yet those who are older and have spent a lifetime trying to serve Jesus, have valuable experiences to share. The older believers in a local church have often been through career struggles, marriage conflicts, and parenting problems. They know the challenges that come from living in a sinful world. Those who are older should look for opportunities to teach or share their lives with younger people. Not engaging in your church removes the opportunity for that to happen.

Negative examples of godliness in older age

The Bible is a realistic book. While we have seen helpful examples of godliness in older age, not all older people are worthy of emulating! For balance, we will look closely at a few ways that our latter years could be misused.

Solomon: A godly start and a terrible finish

Soon after Solomon was crowned king of Israel, he showed his devotion to his God. He loved the Lord, made extraordinary amounts of sacrifices, and asked for wisdom when God said he could have anything he wanted.[26] The early part of Solomon's reign was marked by wise ruling and a growing reputation. He made wise judgements when faced with individual legal problems.[27] He set up wise structures for governing a diverse and tribal kingdom.[28] Solomon was a greatly loved king whose policies benefitted everyone and not only his court. He built the temple and commissioned it; the prayer he spoke upon the dedication of the temple was remarkable for its understanding of God and human nature.[29] Solomon's wealth and wisdom were known internationally.[30]

This does not mean that Solomon was perfect. There were hints even in his early rule that he was allied too closely to Egypt, for example.[31] Despite this, the report of his reign from 1 Kings 2-10 is almost entirely positive. Solomon ruled over the golden age of Israel; this was the peak of the kingdom's wealth and power. When we get to 1 Kings 11, it is a terrible shock for us to hear how he moved away from faithfulness to the true God in his later years. The writer of 1 Kings told us of his many wives and concubines from other nations; marriage alliances made for political and romantic reasons. Other than leading to massive scheduling problems, these marriages led to this:

> *For when Solomon was old his wives turned away his heart after other gods, and his heart was not wholly true to the LORD his God, as was the heart of David his father.*
>
> *(1 Kings 11:4)*

Solomon, the great and faithful king, ended his reign building temples to other gods like Ashtoreth and Chemosh! This was not just to appease his wives, though it might have started this way. The verse above points out that his heart turned away from the true God to other gods. He personally worshipped these other gods; these other temples were not only for his wives to use. This is a sad example of a faithful life diverted into idolatry towards the end.

None of us wants to end up this way. I am sure Solomon never envisaged this either! But step by step, small concession by small concession, we can start to shift away from our faithfulness to God over time. We can chase comfort and the finer things in life later in our working years. We can overemphasize the importance of family and drop the godly habit of Bible reading we once had. Down the track, in our retirement years, we can end up a long way from where we started. If we are not careful, the things of this world can become what matters most to us. Solomon is a sobering example; if it happened to him, it could happen to anyone.

Christians should be growing in godliness and knowledge of God over time. Don't assume that you will do this; you need to put in conscious effort to maintain faithfulness. Resist the call to selfishness that retirement shouts to you. There are better ways to spend your later years than in the worship of comfort and possessions and experiences, those false gods that are never enough.

Hezekiah: Selfishness later in life

If you read the history of the kings of Judah, you will find a great many evil kings. There were kings that completely rejected the true God and worshipped the Canaanite gods. Some kings came to power by killing the previous king. Compared to these rulers, King Hezekiah was a wonderful king. His father Ahaz burned his own son as an offering to another god,[32] so the fact that he was a good and faithful king after such a parental example is remarkable. Hezekiah also reigned through the fall of the northern kingdom and the siege of Jerusalem, so there were many external pressures on him and many tough decisions to be made.

Hezekiah was a faithful king, doing what was right in the eyes of the Lord.[33] He removed the high places where his people made sacrifices to other gods; this would have been an unpopular move with his people, but he chose to do what was right. He humbled himself when faced with the threat of the Assyrians, and he listened to the word of the prophet Isaiah.[34] The assessment of his rule by the writer of 2 Kings is glowing:

> [5]*He trusted in the LORD, the God of Israel, so that there was none like him among all the kings of*

Judah after him, nor among those who were before him. ⁶For he held fast to the LORD. He did not depart from following him, but kept the commandments that the LORD commanded Moses.

(2 Kings 18:5-6)

Considering all that he faced and the family he came from, it may seem odd to include Hezekiah in this list of bad examples. The reason for his inclusion is because of something that happened late in his reign. Hezekiah received envoys from a nation named Babylon. He showed these envoys all the treasures of Judah and the temple, which was incredibly foolish. Isaiah the prophet told Hezekiah that Babylon would destroy all the wealth of his kingdom and take the king's children and castrate them. This shocking news was met with a surprising response:

Then Hezekiah said to Isaiah, "The word of the LORD that you have spoken is good." For he thought, "Why not, if there will be peace and security in my days?"

(2 Kings 20:19)

Good? This word from the Lord is good? That his children will be castrated and serve another king and the kingdom would fall? This is a complete tragedy! The reason Hezekiah thought it was good was because there would be peace and security for him personally while he lived. This tragedy would be a problem for the next generation. As it's not his problem, he doesn't need to worry about it.

What a horrible response from a generally godly king! This is something we should take as a warning. We must not become so selfish later in life that we lose interest in the problems that face the church or the next generation. It is probable that issues will come up in the church that threaten unity or growth. If this is our church family, our response must be, 'What can I do to help?' I pray that none of us uses the fact that an issue doesn't directly impact us as a reason to avoid contributing to assist others. We are still part of the church family, even when we are older, which means we hurt when others are hurting.[35]

The king from Ecclesiastes 4: Failing to listen

Among the many useful things the Teacher of Ecclesiastes has to teach us is the example of the old and foolish king. There is no evidence that this was referring to a real king, though I am sure many kings in world history would fit the description! The example we are given is this:

> [13]*Better was a poor and wise youth than an old and foolish king who no longer knew how to take advice.* [14]*For he went from prison to the throne, though in his own kingdom he had been born poor.* [15]*I saw all the living who move about under the sun, along with that youth who was to stand in the king's place.* [16]*There was no end of all the people, all of whom he led. Yet those who come later will not rejoice in him. Surely this also is vanity and a striving after wind.*
>
> *(Ecclesiastes 4:13-16)*

The king of this passage had risen from the ranks of the poor, even from prison, to become the king. While this kind of progression is more possible today, no king came from such humble backgrounds in the ancient world. This king would be an extremely capable person who had achieved a great deal. He ruled over a large nation. Yet, in the end, his rule would not be celebrated or remembered with fondness after his death. He was better as a poor and wise youth than he was as an older, powerful man. Why? In his old age, he became foolish because he no longer knew how to take advice.

That phrase "no longer" suggests that age and achievement had changed this man. Once he quickly took advice; that was part of what made him wise in the first place. Now, as an old man, he no longer listened to what others had to say. He had power and past achievements; he had become proud and no longer listened as he once did.

We have seen that wisdom does often increase with age and experience. However, it is not always this way. Age can bring about pride instead. Someone who has all they need and much of what they want can feel that they can stop learning. They might stop reading and thinking and evaluating their worldview. They might be resistant to any change, thinking that what they are used to is better than any alternatives. However wise and experienced such a person is, they cause all kinds of problems for those around them. To use the words of the Teacher of Ecclesiastes, no-one will rejoice at their memory after they have gone! We must never be so proud that we cannot learn more and listen to those around us. Nobody has full knowledge of all things in this life. We can always learn and grow. We must be a blessing to others, not a reason to make their lives more difficult.

What can we conclude about the examples we have seen?

Age and wisdom tend to go together, but they don't have to! We are sinful people, and we are tempted towards selfishness at every stage of our lives. Just because someone has more life experience or has made many wise decisions in the past does not mean they will always act that way. Solomon and Hezekiah are warnings that we might turn from God or from compassion for God's people at the end of a lifetime of faithfulness. We must be on our guard.

It is possible to remain faithful and work on godliness all of our lives. Moses was a sinner, sure, but he did what was asked of him throughout his long life. Joshua and Caleb were vigorous men even into very old age, inspiring those around them and encouraging them to faithfulness. Samuel was consistently faithful in his service of God and treatment of others, despite living a very public life that everyone could observe. Keep at it. Having faithful older believers in a church is a blessing beyond counting. Like the Biblical examples in this chapter, those struggling with following Jesus need people to look up to, people who have been there before. People who are still actively striving for godliness. We all need to know it can be done and what faithfulness in older age looks like. Perhaps you could be that example others need?

Many of us are uncomfortable with the idea of being an example. Yes, being older doesn't in itself mean we worthy of emulation. We should strive, however, to be someone worth respecting and listening to. That is possible for all older Christians. If that is not you right now, if you find you are excessively proud and have fallen into the trap of that old king of Ecclesiastes 4, do something about it. Spend time in prayer confessing this to God and work hard on listening to others. If you are convicted that you love comfort and respect too much and have not spent the effort on godliness you should have, there is time to work on that too. If you have drifted into inactivity and detachment from your church family, look for ways to become more involved or ask your pastor how you can serve. Be that example the younger people around you need.

Too many older Christians use their age or retired status as an excuse not to serve God. The positive Biblical examples we have seen were not like that. God, in His wisdom, has used very old people like Abraham and Moses in his work. These were older people with flaws, and in the case of Moses, even older people who initially didn't want to serve as God called them to! Yet they served well to God's glory and remain an example to us today. Of course, being older does mean specific challenges like reduced energy and possibly health problems, which we will look at directly in later chapters. What matters is our attitude and intention. We should be considering how we can serve God in the situation we find ourselves today. Don't use age as an excuse. Retirement from work doesn't mean retirement from the service of God. Use your age and experience well for God's glory and to build up God's church.

Chapter 8
Seeking the kingdom first in older age

Our perspective changes a great deal depending on where we are standing. A mountain range might look like tiny triangles from a great distance yet seem an overwhelming mass from closer up. Likewise, our perspective on central teachings from the Bible can change as we grow older. It's not that the Bible teaches different principles; they just apply differently to older people instead of younger people.

One of the great blessings of the Bible is that it is useful for everyone, regardless of age. In this chapter, we will look at some fundamental Biblical principles that, while they are not written explicitly with older people in mind, have a lot to say to older people and should change how we think about retirement.

Seek the kingdom first

In the Sermon on the Mount from Matthew 5 to 7, Jesus outlines what it looks like to live as a disciple. Once we have understood how much Jesus has done for us, we should work hard to live a life worthy of one who has been saved. One of the most challenging passages in this section of Matthew is this:

> *25"Therefore I tell you, do not be anxious about your life, what you will eat or what you will drink, nor about your body, what you will put on. Is not life more than food, and the body more than clothing? 26Look at the birds of the air: they neither sow nor reap nor gather into barns, and yet your heavenly Father feeds them. Are you not of more value than they? 27And which of you by being anxious can add a single hour to his span of life? 28And why are you anxious about clothing?*

Consider the lilies of the field, how they grow: they neither toil nor spin, ²⁹yet I tell you, even Solomon in all his glory was not arrayed like one of these. ³⁰But if God so clothes the grass of the field, which today is alive and tomorrow is thrown into the oven, will he not much more clothe you, O you of little faith? ³¹Therefore do not be anxious, saying, 'What shall we eat?' or 'What shall we drink?' or 'What shall we wear?' ³²For the Gentiles seek after all these things, and your heavenly Father knows that you need them all. ³³But seek first the kingdom of God and his righteousness, and all these things will be added to you. ³⁴Therefore do not be anxious about tomorrow, for tomorrow will be anxious for itself. Sufficient for the day is its own trouble."

(Matthew 6:25-7:1)

A younger person reading this, full of enthusiasm, may read v33 and aim to do great things for God with their lives. Perhaps this will inspire them to vocational ministry or a life focussed on God instead of other things. A person who has been a Christian for a long time may read the same verse and assume they already do this adequately, rather than thinking hard about how to apply it. That's the problem with most familiar Bible passages; we get so used to them we don't feel the impact that the dramatic counter-cultural instructions should have.

Seeking the kingdom of God and his righteousness is a command for all times in our lives. There is no exemption clause in Matthew 6:33 for those who are retired. I argue that the challenge of seeking God first instead of what to eat or drink or wear is a more significant issue for those who are in the latter stages of life. You likely have more money and nicer things when you are older than when you were a young adult. The more things you have, the more comfort you enjoy, the harder it is to seek God first. We can withdraw into our comfortable houses, head off on regular pleasant holidays, and dream mainly of trying that new restaurant or enjoying an afternoon in the shed. That's how everyone else who doesn't know Jesus lives. Christians are called to more than that. We need to ask first how we can serve God first with our lives, not how we can serve ourselves first and possibly find some time for God if we have any left over.

Some retirees, of course, will not be wealthy. There will be many who live on a modest pension and need to be careful with the money they have. This passage also speaks to those in this situation. Don't be anxious about tomorrow and don't fall into the trap of being bitter if this is your situation. Riches in this life are not an expectation; we should focus on the riches awaiting us in heaven and praise God for his generosity to us. Even if there is reason to be anxious, remember that you have a God who loves you. You need to look to serve Jesus first. Finances can take as prominent a position in the minds of those who are poor as it does in those who are rich; the poor worry about having enough, and the rich worry about keeping it. Whether wealthy or struggling, the command to seek Jesus first applies to all Christians. Don't live for other things. Jesus matters more.

Don't add caveats to clear Bible teaching

The Bible is full of radical commands. We are told to

love the Lord our God with all our heart, soul, mind and strength.[1] We are called to love our neighbour as ourselves.[2] Christians cannot serve God and money.[3] Husbands are to love their wives more than their own bodies.[4] Believers are told to take radical action to deal with anything that leads them into sin.[5] We are to love Jesus more than our physical families.[6] We are to hold to following Jesus even if persecution and death are possibilities.[7]

It is tempting to add some kind of caveat or 'escape clause' to these commands to soften the impact and make it easier on us. This is not just a problem for older people! We know we cannot serve both God and money, but most of us give it a try anyway. We know we should love our wives, but if they are not easy to love right now, well then, we think we can ignore that one unless they change their attitude.

God requires obedience. If you are a retiree or someone who is getting older, there is a strong temptation to use your age or limitations as an easy excuse to avoid these commands. We start to think to ourselves: "Yes, I know I should love my neighbour as myself. But I don't have the energy I once did. Frankly, it is hard enough looking after myself and surely someone else can do it". We can talk ourselves out of radical service. In the end, we run the danger of looking like everyone else who does not know Jesus.

A Christian life should be a life that is radically different from the life of someone who is not Christian. We should be like salt that is readily noticeable as present in even a large meal. God does not expect those who are 70 to serve him in the same way as someone who is 21! But God does expect radical faithfulness that is appropriate to whatever stage of life you are currently in. For an older person, loving your neighbour might mean offering prayer and a phone call rather than rushing over with a hot meal. Choosing to serve God instead of money might mean intentionally having one less holiday in order to support that young ministry apprentice at your church. There is always a way you can make decisions that are different from non-Christians for the sake of the gospel.

Don't use your age as an excuse. Look honestly at your circumstances and choose to live a life that looks different from other retirees for the sake of the gospel.

Your identity in Christ is the same whether old or young

We often measure someone's worth by what they can contribute to society. Young people usually have the energy to work, get involved in church, and keep up with friends or a young family. Those who are elderly can look at those active people with longing; they used to be able to do that. Age often brings limitations in energy and possibly health, and many start to think that they are worth less because of this.

If that's you, the gospel is excellent news indeed! Paul puts it this way:

> *There is neither Jew nor Greek, there is neither slave nor free, there is no male and female, for you are all one in Christ Jesus.*
>
> *(Galatians 3:28)*

I think it would be fair to extend this to include: there

is neither young nor old, for you are all one in Christ Jesus. This doesn't mean that there are no differences between young people and older people. It means that every Christian is equal in Christ Jesus. None of us is saved by what we do. Young, energetic people are saved by Jesus' death in their place. Older people are also saved by Jesus' death in their place. God doesn't rank people based on what they can contribute to society or the church. Every Christian is of infinite value to God; he sent his own Son to die in their place.

Society might well imply that older people are worth less than young people. God doesn't measure people that way. If you are a Christian, you are immensely valuable. You are part of God's family. You are perfect in God's sight.

Understanding this can change your whole outlook on the world. You don't need to live up to what the younger people around you do. You are already deeply loved by God. That gives you security and worth that no one can take away.

But I am no-one special!

Many of the examples of the previous chapter were taken from great leaders in Biblical times. As helpful as those examples are, perhaps you think that these people belong in a different category to yourself. You might not be a senior Christian leader or pastor. You most likely have not been tasked by God to defeat some country or breach an enemy city's defences. I would be somewhat surprised if three strange men had promised that you would have a child when aged in your nineties! If we are just ordinary people, no-one special, how can we be examples for others or be used mightily by God in our latter years?

Most of us won't fill stadiums like Billy Graham. And that's fine. We read about people like Moses and Samuel and Caleb, and we think that all faithful believers have to be prominent leaders. That's not true. In the time of these great leaders, there were also a great many faithful ordinary people, serving God and obeying his commandments as best they could in their circumstances. Their stories are generally not recorded for us in the Bible, but we can be sure they were there. Even in the dark days of King Ahab, God told the prophet Elijah that there were seven thousand people who were faithful and had not bowed down to Baal.[8] Many people simply strived to serve God through ethical business practices, an attempt at a godly family life, and through serving others in their local community. God's world doesn't just need pastors; it needs faithful workers, godly young mothers, and even retirees who seek the kingdom of God first.

Don't compare yourself to the most prominent Christian leader you know. That can make us a little defeatist, thinking that we cannot do anything if we cannot be like them. Think about how you can serve Jesus in your context. The question facing all of us is: "How can I serve Jesus best today?". Maybe the best way to use your time today is to spend time in prayer. Perhaps a visit to someone stuck at home or hospital will be a great encouragement. There is always something that can be done to serve Jesus better.

Redeeming the time

Time is a limited resource. At various times, the Biblical writers encourage us to redeem the time.[9] We should be careful how we use the time we have.

A significant advantage of being retired or working less is that you do have more time. Young people are pushed hard in their education, young people are often juggling a job and the challenges of young children, and those in middle age have an often all-encompassing career together with raising teenagers and helping elderly relatives. Almost everyone you will ever meet will tell you that they are busy.

The difference with those who are retired is that they have more control over their time. Sure, most retirees I know are busy too. Retirees can always find things to do, but they are not beholden to a boss like they once were. They get to choose what to do and who to do it with. With this freedom comes responsibility. What is a good way to spend time if you are a retired person? How can you best structure your week?

Again, the best way to frame this is to ask how your use of time honours King Jesus. If all of your time and effort is spent on hobbies and friends, don't even pagans do that? Christians should be distinctive in how they spend their extra time in retirement. It has to include more time in prayer. It should involve using gifts to serve the local church. There may be all kinds of opportunities to serve Jesus, some of which we will explore later in this book.

Don't just let your time fill up without thinking. If you do that, your time will naturally fill up only with self-satisfying activities. Christians need to be more strategic than this. God has given you extra time; what will you do with what you have been given? When you stand before God in glory, will you be pleased to present what you have done with your talents to him? If all you have to show for a few decades of time you control is a low golf handicap, stamps in a passport, and beautiful paintings you have made, is that enough?

Please don't mishear me here. There is nothing wrong with attending a craft group if you enjoy craft. Playing golf and going on a cruise are not sins! There is a time for rest, and God didn't make us to work non-stop. What I am suggesting here is that retirement must be more than just hobbies and recreation for Christians. Actively plan to serve Jesus, else you might wake up one day and realise you have spent all the time you have been given only on serving yourself.

Consider ministry and mission as an option

We live in a world where many have not heard the gospel. All Christians should be involved in the work of ministry in some form, but some people decide to devote their lives to ministry as a vocation. Many of the missionaries who are sent overseas and many of the pastors who graduate from theological college are younger instead of older.

Let's not limit ourselves. Those who are older are uniquely placed to consider ministry and mission work as an option.

Yes, young ministry candidates may have the enthusiasm and the energy that comes with that age. They also can devote themselves to potentially many decades in ministry or on the mission field. Retirees might not have the same energy and drive. However, they have advantages that younger people do not: experience and time. If you have been involved in a good church, learning from faithful teaching and serving as you are able, your theology and understanding of the Bible will be strong. Your life situation might also be less complicated as you no longer need to consider a work-life balance. You should ask: might I be used to serve Jesus in a more extensive way, even now?

I know of quite a number of retirees who are active in ministry or mission service. Our church recently decided to support a middle-aged couple who are heading to South America after several decades of pastoral ministry at home. One widow I know is still extremely active in women's ministry in her local church. A couple I know decided to self-fund a move to another country to encourage ministry work there.

You don't need to move countries to do ministry! There are many older Christians who help run Bible studies for seniors or who co-ordinate visiting of sick or lonely church members. Some older people have been able to serve wholeheartedly as elders or deacons in their churches, which they previously did not have the time to do. The extra time retirement gives provides opportunities many have never had open to them before.

Conclusion: The honest application of the Bible

God calls us all, young and old, to radical discipleship in the pages of the Bible. We are to love God with all our heart, mind, soul and strength. We are to love our neighbours as ourselves. We are to use whatever God gives us for the work of his kingdom, as explained in the parable of the talents [10]. None of these commands is restricted to the young. We must not add in our own loopholes, assuming only younger people can do these things while we end up living selfish lives like those who don't know Jesus.

Whatever our age and limitations, we should ask how we can best serve God with what he has given to us. Retirement gives people unique opportunities in terms of time and experience to serve Jesus with. Let's use our time well. We all look forward to the day when the Father welcomes us with "Well done, good and faithful servant. Enter into your master's happiness".[11] Even if that day seems closer than it once did, let's keep on striving to finish well.

Section 3
Practical challenges retirement poses

Chapter 9
Fighting the urge to criticise change and idolise the 'good old days'

No one really likes change, no matter how old we are. We all find a routine and lifestyle that is comfortable for us, and once we have that, we hold onto it for as long as we can. As the saying goes, the only person who likes change is a baby with a wet nappy! Most of us tend to fall into the same kind of routine week by week, doing the same sort of things, visiting the same types of places, with occasional breaks of routine due to holidays.

The older we get, the more fixed our routines seem to be. Although this is a generalisation and not true of everyone, older people tend to like things to stay the same as they always have been. Older people are less likely to be interested in changing their clothes to follow the latest fashion or in exploring new music styles. The houses of retirees are more likely to be full of items of a sentimental nature rather than furnished with the newest style.

There is nothing wrong with liking routine and preferring things to stay the same; I like those things too! The problem is that the culture shifts even though our preferences do not. In every generation, older people complain about the behaviour and lifestyle of younger people. Indeed, Socrates said this about the youth of ancient Greece:

"The children now love luxury; they have bad manners, contempt for authority; they show disrespect for elders and love chatter in place of exercise. Children are now tyrants, not the servants of their households. They no longer rise when elders enter the room. They contradict their parents, chatter before company, gobble up dainties at the table, cross their legs, and tyrannize their teachers.".[1]

It is natural for older people today to fall into the same kind of outlook, complaining about how culture has changed and constantly being critical of younger people. A cursory glance of the letters to the editor of any major newspaper will reveal this attitude is alive and well! We can assume that the way we prefer to live is the correct way and that everyone younger is wrong because they live differently.

This attitude can seep into the local church too. Many churches contain a significant proportion of older believers who have faithfully supported and served in that church for many decades. They love Jesus and have things running the way that they prefer them to be. Through God's providence, however, the demographics of churches can change. Younger people might start to attend the church. The children of the young families begin to grow up and ask for new ministries or for the worship style to be different. The leadership might hire a younger pastor to bring in new energy and ideas, leading to proposals to start new ministries or head in a different strategic direction.

What do you think the older believers in a church like this are tempted to do? There is often a strong pull to resist any attempt at change. Change in worship style might mean accepting different instruments and learning new songs. New outreach ministries might mean interaction with people very different to you. These things are tricky for anyone but especially for many older people. It is easy to immediately reject all change as wrong and to refuse to compromise on anything. That will lead to either the younger people leaving (which no one wants) or the church setting up one service for older people and one service for young people (which is a poor expression of the unity we have in Christ). There needs to be a better way than this.

The good old days might not have been that good

If you browse through anyone's photo albums, you will notice something interesting. They are full of good times. We love to preserve the memories of holidays, birthday parties and babies taking their first steps. If all we had to remember the past was our photo albums, we would have a false impression of what really happened. So much of our past lives were routine and not worthy of having a photo taken. And there were terrible times, too; most people don't want to preserve images of tears at a funeral or frustration at losing a job.

Just like our photos, our memories can be selective. When enough time has passed, it is usually possible to look back on our past with fondness. We filter out the painful and negative things and instead recall the positive things. We start to reminisce about the 'good old days' when things were better than they are now. Using that perspective, everything today seems somehow worse than it was when we were younger.

The 'good old days' were rarely as good as we remember them to be. Compared to fifty years ago, our world is wildly different. It is easy to notice the things that are worse: vast numbers of people addicted to social media or the rise of internet pornography, for example. But it's not all worse. Cars are now cheaper and much safer. There have been great strides forward towards equal treatment of men and women. The life expectancy in much of the world has increased by many years. We can communicate with loved ones all over the globe with ease.

Hans Rosling explained this very well in his enlightening book 'Factfulness'.[2] We all tend to have a dim view of the world based on what we see on the news. The reality is quite different. On many objective measures, the world is better today than it was in the past. There are fewer people in abject poverty. The gap between rich and poor is smaller. The education levels around the world are higher. Significantly higher vaccination rates mean much less serious disease. The world is getting better in many ways; the old is not always better than the new.

Once more, the Teacher of Ecclesiastes has something to say about this point:

> *Say not, "Why were the former days better than these?" For it is not from wisdom that you ask this.*
>
> *(Ecclesiastes 7:10)*

The point the Teacher is making here is not that the current days are better than the former days. His point is that comparing the past to the present is unwise; it does not lead anywhere useful. All that romanticising the past can bring is dissatisfaction with the present.

Fond selective memories of the past are not a modern phenomenon. The people of Israel in the wilderness thousands of years ago fell into the same trap. They had been rescued from the oppression of slavery in Egypt, where they cried for rescue[3] and suffered the genocide of their children.[4] God showed them his power and rescued them through the plagues and the parting of the sea. He fed them with bread that fell from the sky each day. By anyone's measure, these people were blessed by God! Yet, even in the midst of being rescued, they looked back on their time in slavery with fondness:

> *⁴Now the rabble that was among them had a strong craving. And the people of Israel also wept again and said, "Oh that we had meat to eat! ⁵We remember the fish we ate in Egypt that cost nothing, the cucumbers, the melons, the leeks, the onions, and the garlic. ⁶But now our strength is dried up, and there is nothing at all but this manna to look at."*
>
> *(Numbers 11:4-6)*

Talk about selective memory! These saved people looked back on their bondage as a time of feasting and plenty. They somehow failed to remember the whips and the making of bread without straw, the unrealistic work quotas, and the systematic murder to reduce their numbers.

There is a time for reminiscing about the 'good old days'. There is nothing wrong with telling stories and fondly remembering what has happened in the past. But don't let that cloud your perception of what is happening today. The new is not always worse than the old; if we're honest, sometimes it is far better.

Jesus' take on old and new

Jesus often engaged with the Pharisees during his earthly ministry. The Pharisees loved tradition. They were careful not only to obey the law of Moses but also to follow the traditions of respected Jewish teachers. This zeal for law-keeping was not only a personal matter; the Pharisees were known as the moral policemen of their day. They were concerned that everyone kept their rules, even when those rules were not directly from the Scriptures.

For example, the Pharisees expected regular fasting from food as part of the spiritual life of all Jewish people. This was a tradition rather than an expectation from the Scriptures. The law of Moses allowed fasting but only prescribed a fast on one day a year, the Day of Atonement. In fact, there were far more feast days in the Biblical calendar than fast days! The rules that the Pharisees created led to conflict with Jesus, as we see in this passage:

> *33And they [the Pharisees and the scribes] said to him, "The disciples of John fast often and offer prayers, and so do the disciples of the Pharisees, but yours eat and drink." 34And Jesus said to them, "Can you make wedding guests fast while the bridegroom is with them? 35The days will come when the bridegroom is taken away from them, and then they will fast in those days." 36He also told them a parable: "No one tears a piece from a new garment and puts it on an old garment. If he does, he will tear the new, and the piece from the new will not match the old. 37And no one puts new wine into old wineskins. If he does, the new wine will burst the skins and it will be spilled, and the skins will be destroyed. 38But new wine must be put into fresh wineskins. 39And no one after drinking old wine desires new, for he says, 'The old is good.'"*
>
> (Luke 5:33-39)

Jesus did not expect his disciples to fast. He was the bridegroom, and his presence was a reason for celebration and not for mourning. Jesus' arrival signified a time of newness and rejoicing for his disciples and all who understood who he was. Fasting was not appropriate or expected in that context.

The parable Jesus used in v36-38 contrasts the old and the new. It makes no sense to cut up new clothes to patch old ones; you will have destroyed both of them. Likewise, new wine would burst old pre-stretched wineskins, destroying the wineskin and spilling the wine. Jesus' point to the Pharisees, and the disciples of John, is clear: he is something new. You cannot just keep your old existing traditions and religion and add Jesus to it. No, true faith is not like that at all. True faith is about understanding how wonderful Jesus is and trusting in Him rather than in traditions. We are only right with God through trusting in Jesus. The Scriptures prepare the way for Jesus, but the way of following Jesus is not through traditions but through faith and rejoicing in Jesus.

Why is this passage relevant to our discussion about change? Older Christians are not in the same situation as the Pharisees. They understand that they are only saved by faith and not law-keeping and tradition. Yet, there is a danger of falling into the same mindset. It is so easy to elevate our traditions, the ways things have always been done, to a higher level than they should have. We must be careful to ensure that we are judging the discipleship of others against the Scriptures and not on what our personal preferences might be.

An important principle: Scripture alone and not tradition

Everyone has traditions, even those who think of themselves as innovative and impulsive. We fall into the same patterns of life. We shop in the same places and take the same route to work or our homes. We eat the same kinds of foods most of the time. There is nothing wrong with liking things to be comfortable and familiar, however we need to beware of holding our traditions so tightly that we are unwilling to change them for good reasons.

One of the key teachings of the Protestant Reformation was 'Sola Scriptura' which means 'by the Scriptures alone'. This means that our ultimate authority is the Word of God. God's word is reliable because it is from God. We should expect the Scriptures to be useful for us, both in a positive way in terms of training and teaching and in a critical way in terms of rebuking and correcting us.[5] We need to allow God's word to dwell in us richly,[6] to meditate on it day and night,[7] and to have our thinking transformed through the renewing of our minds.[8]

If we hold to the Bible being the ultimate authority for us, this will mean many things will be non-negotiable when it comes to church. We will want to make sure that the good news about Jesus remains central to all we do. We will want to speak strongly against sin and call people to repentance. We will want to hear the Bible faithfully explained and applied in all kinds of ways. Whatever our age, we need to remain firm on the core teaching of the Bible. That is not negotiable. How we apply these principles, and to what extent we allow tradition to guide our practice, will be a matter of wisdom that different generations might disagree about.

In the end, we need to remember this critical point: **our personal preferences may well not be the same as what the Bible says**. As we get older, and start to be more set in the habits we have built up over time, we need to remember that our preferences are not more important than Scripture. I grew up in a church that only used the organ for accompanying songs. The prevailing opinion was that pianos and guitars were inferior and unsuitable for music in a worship service. This was a strongly held view that was expressed in many a congregational meeting! Yet there is no Biblical basis for it at all. The organ may well be appropriate for musical accompaniment, but there is no verse hidden anywhere that says the organ is the only suitable instrument! There comes a time we need to step back and slow down a moment; just because something is different to how we've always done it does not mean it is wrong. It might be wrong, it might be correct, but it needs to be weighed against Scripture.

We can find another example in what people wear to church. In previous generations, and in certain cultures today, it is expected that men wear suits or at least jackets and women wear dresses and perhaps hats. People had a set of clothes kept aside for 'Sunday best' which were not worn anywhere else. The intent was to express a sense of reverence that was appropriate for the occasion. In some cultures and among younger people, the dress code for church is far more casual. What people wear has always changed from generation to generation. When others feel differently from you about what is appropriate to wear to church, it doesn't mean that we are right and they are irreverent and wrong. The Bible is silent on what we should wear to a church gathering, so we shouldn't make this a significant point of conflict.[9] What we prefer and what the Bible says are not the same thing.

Please don't mishear me here. I am not saying that traditions should be easily cast away and that the younger generations should always get their way when there is a conflict! In many cases, traditions have been formed over time for good reasons. Any plans to change traditions and habits should involve both sides explaining their perspective. As the older generations often hold more positions of authority in the church, retirees must be careful not to squash any genuine attempt to reform the church's practice to better match the Bible and better reach the culture.

Being more open to something new

Being open to new ways of doing things sounds like a good idea in theory but it is hard to do in practice. When a younger person thinks about music and dress and evangelism and all kinds of other things differently to what we do, the knee-jerk reaction is often to think they are wrong. We have been around for longer than they have. There are good reasons to do things in a certain way.

How do we curb this impulse to avoid change? We need to take a deep breath and think through the issues honestly and slowly. Our first reaction might not be the most godly or helpful one. We need to remember that our world desperately needs to hear the good news about Jesus. We also need to understand that the broader culture is constantly changing. Previous evangelistic programmes that relied on people with some basic church or Sunday School background won't work now when that experience doesn't apply to most people. We need to engage with a broader range of cultures and understand their thinking and religions more than was the case decades ago. The rise of the internet and social media gives us opportunities for the gospel and raises challenges we would never have thought of. For all these reasons and more, we need to be open to changing how we operate as Christians and churches.

Ideally, a local church should consist of young people and old people and everyone in-between. That will mean compromise and change. Every church has had to decide how to deliver its music program. We want the worship service to be helpful for older believers and for teenagers. That will mean, at times, being open to creativity and change. It will mean involving younger people in ministry who approach it differently from how we might do things. In the end, being in a church that contains young and old is a blessing for both. We need both enthusiasm and experience. We need a sense of creativity as well as an understanding of tradition. In the end, we are stronger together, and we need to take the time to understand that change might be required for the sake of the gospel.

We live in a culture where everyone loves to complain and criticise. So many letters to the editor and internet posts simply complain about how society is. We can find ourselves becoming bitter and inflexible. Younger people in the church may then view the older people as those who care more for tradition than for the Bible. There is a better way than this. Look for opportunities to encourage others. Come to church on a Sunday morning having prayed that you will be able to build people up today. When you see a younger person attempting some new ministry or initiative, write them an encouraging note or tell them of your appreciation in person. Look for the good instead of focussing on the loss of tradition and comfort that might come through this new ministry.

Let's aim to have the attitude of Paul, who was creative in his attempts to save some.[10] Change is always hard, especially in churches. Let's be Bible people who judge everything against the Scriptures and don't assume the way we do it now is the best way. By God's grace, we will grow in our thinking and faith as we assess everything fairly. All believers, old and young, should want the same thing: to see Jesus glorified. If we work at encouraging first rather than criticising, we will be one step closer to seeing that happen.

Chapter 10
Serving Jesus despite loss of energy, disability, and other limitations

As much as we might imagine an active and happy retirement, older age does sometimes bring health challenges along with it. This could mean minor concerns like having less energy than you once did and sore joints in the morning. For some people, however, health problems will have a much more significant impact on their lives. Some will cope with lung or heart conditions; others will have to navigate what life looks like managing diabetes or the after-effects of a stroke. There may even come a time when we require extra assistance with everyday tasks or have to move into some kind of residential care facility.

How should Christians think about the health problems that are likely to become more of an issue post-retirement? It is easy to become somewhat bitter and frustrated at life. Knowing what you could do at one time and realising this will not be possible again creates a loss that we will mourn. We need to have a realistic view of our latter years, but this does not mean we should end up angry and bitter. Whether physically fit or severely limited due to our health, we should be seeking the kingdom of God first.

How is this possible? As usual, it is a good idea to see what God has to say about these things in the Bible.

The Bible is not sentimental; it describes ageing and its impact

Many who have never read the Bible imagine it to be full of pious, perfect people who live flawless lives for us to follow. The reality is quite the opposite. God's word describes a world that is imperfect, full of imperfect people. We do not read some kind of sanitised view of life with the tricky bits glossed over or ignored; we read about real life with all its challenges and difficulties. So, when it comes to describing what it is like to be old, the Bible doesn't hold back. The Bible does not pretend that getting older is easy.

Many of the older people in the Bible have some kind of struggle with their health. The prophet Ahijah met Jeroboam alone in an open field in his younger days,[1] but in his latter days, he was restricted to his house because "his eyes were dim because of his age".[2] Eli the priest also lost his eyesight in his old age and became a man who spent significant time seated because he was "old and heavy".[3] King Asa of Judah served God faithfully for many years, but "in his old age he was diseased in his feet".[4] Age takes its toll on everyone.

Barzillai the Gileadite, who has possibly the best name in the whole Bible, expresses what it is like to be old in a most memorable way. Barzillai helped David when he was on the run from Absalom by providing supplies for his journey. When David returned, he invited Barzillai to join him in Jerusalem, where he would be cared for in the royal court as a reward for his service. Barzillai replied with these words:

> [34]*But Barzillai said to the king, "How many years have I still to live, that I should go up with the king to Jerusalem?* [35]*I am this day eighty years old. Can I discern what is pleasant and what is not? Can your servant taste what he eats or what he drinks? Can I still listen to the voice of singing men and singing women? Why then should your servant be an added burden to my lord the king?"*
> *(2 Samuel 19:34-35)*

That's an honest answer! In his old age, Barzillai has lost his sense of taste. He cannot hear the way he once did. He can no longer appreciate the finer things in life. Old age is not glamorous, and it brings fading abilities and growing health problems. Even the healthiest and strongest person will eventually encounter struggles with slowing down as they grow older.

The poem on ageing from Ecclesiastes 12 is likewise honest and memorable:

> *Remember also your Creator in the days of your youth, before the evil days come and the years draw near of which you will say, "I have no pleasure in them"; [2]before the sun and the light and the moon and the stars are darkened and the clouds return after the rain, [3]in the day when the keepers of the house tremble, and the strong men are bent, and the grinders cease because they are few, and those who look through the windows are dimmed, [4]and the doors on the street are shut – when the sound of the grinding is low, and one rises up at the sound of a bird, and all the daughters of song are brought low – [5]they are afraid also of what is high, and terrors are in the way; the almond tree blossoms, the grasshopper drags itself along, and desire fails, because man is going to his eternal home, and the mourners go about the streets – [6]before the silver cord is snapped, or the golden bowl is broken, or the pitcher is shattered at the fountain, or the wheel broken at the cistern, [7]and the dust returns to the earth as it was, and the spirit returns to God who gave it. [8]Vanity of vanities, says the Preacher; all is vanity.*
>
> (Ecclesiastes 12:1-8)

This is a beautiful piece of poetry describing the challenges of old age. The first part of the poem describes the days where youthful pleasures are gone. This is a very clever bit of poetry; it reads literally, but the deeper meaning is obvious if you think a little about it. Verse 2 speaks of the coming darkness, when the sun and light and moon and stars are darkened, a time when the clouds roll in. This also describes the dusk of life, when things are not as vivid as they once were, where darkness is starting to come.

The overriding image of v3-4 is a grand old house that was once impressive but now has fallen into decay. The various pieces of imagery in these verses correspond to body parts and their decline over time. The keepers of the house – the arms – tremble. The strong men – the legs – are bent. Grinders – the teeth – cease, for they are few. Those who look through the windows – the eyes – are dimmed. The doors on the street – the ears – are shut. What once was so impressive has faded. It is recognisable but not what it used to be.

Verse 4b expands a little on the situation. In later life, sounds are interpreted differently; on the one hand, impaired hearing makes ordinary sounds low, but the sound of a bird rouses an older person from sleep. It is true, from what my older friends tell me; most of them are up early with the birds and have lost the ability to sleep in that they once had. With older age also comes fear (v5): fear of heights and fear of jostling in the street. Almond tree blossoms are white; this is speaking of white hair. Grasshoppers usually fly; when we see them drag themselves along, we know they are old. And the fall of desire is speaking of sexual libido; not as obviously in English, but clear in Hebrew. As we read at the end of v5, all of these changes happen because man is going to his eternal home. Mourners are in the streets; friends pass away. Death is near. In that context, the Teacher of Ecclesiastes encourages his readers to remember their God before it is too late and the ageing process finishes in death.

As we have seen elsewhere, the Bible does not view the ageing process through rose-coloured glasses. Ageing brings health problems, slowing down, and being unable to do what you once could. That is the reality of life after the Fall. This is a natural process that we need not be ashamed of or embarrassed about. We will all grow old.

This surely means that we also should have a realistic understanding of our abilities in our later years. We don't need to keep up with the younger ones to have significance. We don't need to hide our wrinkles or our greying or thinning hair. Vanity should not get the better of us.

You are not worth any less to God because you cannot do what you once did. We too easily measure ourselves against the young and beautiful people of the world, or even against our own younger selves. That's not realistic. Remember that you are important in God's sight because of what Jesus did for you. It is not because of what you can do. It is not because of the thickness of your hair or the speed you can walk. You remain of infinite worth to God even when you are not physically what you used to be.

God loves to use the weak to shame the strong

It is a natural thing for us to honour those who are strong and young. Olympic athletes grace the covers of magazines, and younger people advertise beauty products. Even in the church, often it is the university student ministry that is prioritised as 'strategic', while ministry to older believers or those with disabilities can be overlooked.

God doesn't value strength the way that we do. In fact, God seems to love using those who are weak for his purposes. We see this all through Scripture. God chose Moses to lead his people out of Egypt, even though he couldn't speak well and didn't want to do it. Jesus chose a ragtag group of men to be his disciples, impetuous men like Peter who were fishermen instead of scholars or aristocrats. Many of the people remembered as having great faith in the gospels are foreigners, women, prostitutes, disabled, or poor.

We might honour the apostle Paul for his tightly reasoned letters in the New Testament, but he was derided for not being very impressive in person[5] and he struggled with a "thorn" problem his whole life. When he asked God to remove this "thorn", God's answer was:

> "My grace is sufficient for you, for my power is made perfect in weakness."
>
> *(2 Corinthians 12:9)*

In the end, Paul realised it was good for him to have his limitations. His problem, whatever it was, was an ongoing struggle that kept him from becoming conceited. God used someone with significant struggles in his life so powerfully to make it clear that the power came from God and not from Paul. In fact, Paul could conclude that it was when he was weak that he was actually strong. He came to depend on God in his hard times instead of himself.

Paul explained God's use of the weak over the strong in another place:

> ²⁶*For consider your calling, brothers: not many of you were wise according to worldly standards, not many were powerful, not many were of noble birth. ²⁷But God chose what is foolish in the world to shame the wise; God chose what is weak in the world to shame the strong; ²⁸God chose what is low and despised in the world, even things that are not, to bring to nothing things that are, ²⁹so that no human being might boast in the presence of God.*
>
> *(1 Corinthians 1:26-29)*

Do you see how freeing Paul's point is here? You don't need to be an impressive strong young person to be used by God. God loves to use people who are weak in the eyes of the world for his purposes. You might be incredibly useful to God, not because of your innate abilities, but because people can see the grace of God working through someone like you. There are few things more encouraging to younger believers than to see older saints who struggle with their health remaining faithful as servants of the Lord Jesus.

But what could I possibly do to serve God in my situation?

Perhaps you are convinced that those who are older or who have health issues should be active in serving God, but you find it hard to picture what that looks like. After all, you might not be able to preach or lead a congregation or head to the mission field. If age and health issues are limiting factors for you, what might your service of Jesus look like?

There are examples all around us in our churches if only we would look. Many older people in churches I have been part of have been incredibly faithful in prayer. Even if you have some limitation that means you cannot leave your house, you can pray. Perhaps God has given you the great opportunity to spend more time in prayer than you ever have before! Don't focus on your limitations; think about your opportunities to serve. A focus on prayer will change you as well as you present your requests to God, reminding you that even in your time of challenge, your Father hears you.

Several retirees I have known have used their extra time and resources well by showing hospitality to others in the church. Inviting others over for meals is a dying tradition for many struggling to balance busy careers with their home lives. Opening your house to others, or taking them with you to a restaurant, can be a great way to show love to other people and encourage them.

With age comes experience and wisdom. Oh yes, I know that even older believers who have been in the church for decades still feel their lack of understanding! But the reality is that if you are older, you most likely have a more robust Bible knowledge and experience of living out your faith than many younger people. Consider how you might use those talents. You could meet regularly with new Christians to read the Bible with them. You could take the opportunity to serve as a Bible study leader or visit others. You can phone people or use email to encourage others. Even with limited energy, there are so many ways you could use what God has given you to benefit others.

If you find yourself with a more severe disability or limitation, even then you can see your situation as an opportunity for service. I have known many Christians with severe disability and chronic diseases to be a magnificent witness to the health staff and doctors who cared for them. If you have carers come to your house to help you with everyday tasks, the way you treat them and interact with them can shine the light of the gospel into their lives. Never underestimate the influence a faithful believer can have on the world around them simply by living a joyful, faithful life in difficult circumstances.

Moving from bitterness to thankfulness

I recently heard an older Christian pastor say that there are too many grumpy old men in the world. I don't think it's only true of men either! Age does bring problems, and those problems can lead us to be difficult and critical people. We can focus on what we have lost and find ourselves wallowing in self-pity. Yes, older age might not have turned out as we expected it to. Yes, we might have some disability and not be able to do what we once did. All that might be true. In the end, focussing on what we cannot do will only lead to bitterness. There is a better way.

The apostle Paul once again gives us helpful advice here:

> *Finally, brothers, whatever is true, whatever is honorable, whatever is just, whatever is pure, whatever is lovely, whatever is commendable, if there is any excellence, if there is anything worthy of praise, think about these things.*
>
> *(Philippians 4:8)*

It is too simplistic to just say 'look on the bright side' when something like a chronic illness dominates your life. It will help us to consider Paul's context. He wrote the letter to the Philippians from jail. He knew full well what a difficult life was like. Yet he urged contentment in all circumstances,[6] rejoicing whatever happens,[7] and thinking about the things worthy of praise! When we suffer an ongoing disability, chronic pain or other severe limitations, negativity can easily dominate our thinking. We need to be reminded that there are still so many good things to think about. We can look outside and understand how beautiful God's creation is.[8] We can recall what God has done for us in Jesus, like redemption, forgiveness of sins, adoption as his children, and we know that these things are still true in our dark days.[9] We can think about the certain hope we have for the future, a time when our struggles now will be no more and all will be perfect.[10] We can rejoice and find comfort that this life is not all there is and look forward to the perfection of heaven. However dark your days might seem, there are always positives to think about if you trust in Jesus.

When I was a university student, there was an older couple in a church I attended. They had a most difficult life. On the surface, it seemed everything that could go wrong for them had gone wrong. They lost their house because they were guarantor for their son who had a drug problem. They suffered chronic health problems themselves. Yet, if you met them, you would never have guessed this. The wife would often say, "Isn't God wonderful?". And she meant it: God was good to them! Even when all these things happened in their lives, they knew that God's kindness mattered more. I haven't seen them for decades now, but their example will stick with me forever.

You don't need to be defeatist when it comes to your age and limitations, even if they are severe. Instead of constantly saying to yourself, "I cannot do anything useful", ask "what can I do in this situation to serve Jesus?" Your witness to those around you of a faithful, contented life in the face of your struggles will have a more significant impact than you can imagine.

Section 4
Living out a godly life in retirement

Chapter 11
Retirement and money

What is the first thing that pops into your head when you hear the word 'retirement'? If you search the internet or bookstores on the topic, it soon becomes clear that it is 'money' that most people link to retirement. If you are not yet retired, you might be wondering how much money you need to save to retire well. If you are retired, the lack of extra income hitting your bank account might make you wonder if what you have will last for long enough.

This is not a financial planning book. Financial concerns are important, and you should plan wisely when it comes to money. But if your main focus concerning retirement is money, I would strongly suggest that you are looking in the wrong direction. As soon as money becomes central to our thinking, we can find ourselves on dangerous ground and serving the wrong Master.[1]

I have deliberately placed this chapter on money towards the end of this book for that reason. We need to think about financial issues and how they relate to retirement, but other matters must be considered first.

Money has a unique way of capturing our hearts and our thinking, which is why Jesus spoke about it so frequently. We need not just to ask if we have enough money; we need to think Biblically about money and possessions to serve God and not just ourselves.

Putting retirement planning in its proper place

The financial services industry tries to encourage us to put more and more money aside for retirement at every opportunity. Typically, the amount recommended for a comfortable retirement in Australia is somewhere in the range of one million dollars.[2] This is a massive amount to accumulate by retirement age, leading the great majority of the population to fear that they will not have enough. Fear is a great motivator. The closer people get to retirement, the more common it is for workers to put every spare cent into their superannuation or retirement fund.

There is something more important from a Christian perspective to think through here. This fear of not having enough can blind us to the fact that retirement planning can make us very self-focused about our resources. In our worry about the future, we can relegate the Biblical commands to be generous and to remember the poor to the back of our minds. After all, what if I don't have enough for my retirement?

Let's be honest. If you are someone who is planning for retirement, you are likely living in a wealthy country. You are likely not in any real danger of starving or being homeless in your later years. You would probably be surprised to realise that you likely have a net wealth that would place you in the top echelon of the world, even if you have a modest income compared to those who live near you.[3] The fear that the financial services industry is trying to instil into you might sound reasonable like all good marketing does, but is not the whole story. Whatever your stage of life, you need to consider how you can use your resources to serve God well in his world. This means that saving it all for yourself and not giving to the church or the poor is not just selfish; it is living as if you were the master instead of Jesus.

Think stewardship and not ownership

When it comes to a Christian view of money, the key idea is this: all that you have is not actually yours. Everything belongs to God. We are not owners of our money and possessions; instead, we are stewards. We are those of whom an account will be demanded. There will come a day when our Lord and Master will ask us to return what He has given to us and will want to know what we have done with it.[4]

Thinking of money as belonging to God changes everything. We drive more safely in a car that we have borrowed from a friend rather than our own car. We know we have to return it and we are keen to return it in good condition. Likewise, God has been gracious to us with the money and possessions we have. God owns all of it, not just the portion we give to the church or to charity.[5]

Even when our working life ends, our responsibility to be stewards of God's possessions does not. Sure, we might have less income, that is true. This is not a license to be selfish and spend all of our money on ourselves. We are still called to be generous. We still need to budget to support the work of the kingdom of God, whether in the local church or through mission work.

I understand that it is a scary thought that we should be generous when our opportunity for making more money has ended. In reality, how we spend our money in retirement is a good gauge of what our heart is like. If we are only too happy to book the next cruise or upgrade the car but grudge a generous regular donation to the church, perhaps we need to do some self-examination. We must not simply hoard wealth for ourselves.[6] Even those on limited retirement incomes surely have a responsibility to be generous.[7] When you face your Creator, would you be happy to show him where you spent your money?

What we can learn from the minimalist movement

Minimalism has gained a lot of popularity in the past few years.[8] This is a movement that encourages people to intentionally live with fewer possessions. It is a strong reaction against the excesses of materialism and there is much to commend it. Many people have come to realise that accumulating more possessions does not tend to make you happier. There is something freeing about stepping off the constant cycle of buying and consumerism.

Some people take minimalism to an extreme. Some have sold their houses and can fit all of their worldly possessions in a suitcase. Others simply choose to clear out the clutter in their homes and intentionally live with less. It is true that most of us have far more clothes than we could ever wear and tie our happiness too closely to the things we own. Buying a new car or mobile phone is unlikely to make us significantly happier, but most of us continue to live as if it will. We also get so attached to our possessions we develop worries and anxiety about them being stolen or losing value.

What does this have to do with money and retirement? A great deal! It is so easy to think that we can measure a good life by looking at our possessions. By retirement age, we may have accumulated a lot. We may live in a lovely house and drive a good car. We may well have the money to buy many of the things we want and fill our homes with nice things. We could, if we chose, indulge in all the best foods and add quality artwork to our walls. We can shrink our lives into obtaining a series of possessions, with shopping and the pursuit of pleasure being our dominant hobbies.

While it might seem harmless to enjoy what you have worked for your whole life, the problem is that we end up looking for happiness in the wrong place. Constantly chasing the next big experience or purchase will not bring the contentment you are seeking.

As the Teacher of Ecclesiastes wrote:

> [7]*I bought male and female slaves, and had slaves who were born in my house. I had also great possessions of herds and flocks, more than any who had been before me in Jerusalem.* [8]*I also gathered for myself silver and gold and the treasure of kings and provinces. I got singers, both men and women, and many concubines, the delight of the sons of man.* [9]*So I became great and surpassed all who were before me in Jerusalem. Also my wisdom remained with me.* [10]*And whatever my eyes desired I did not keep from them. I kept my heart from no pleasure, for my heart found pleasure in all my toil, and this was my reward for all my toil.* [11]*Then I considered all that my hands had done and the toil I had expended in doing it, and behold, all was vanity and a striving after wind, and there was nothing to be gained under the sun.*
>
> *(Ecclesiastes 2:7-11)*

The Teacher is concluding something similar to what the modern minimalist movement has noted: possessions don't deliver what they promise. We will never achieve purpose and contentment by having enough things. In the end, it is like striving to catch the wind (v11); all our efforts to accumulate possessions end up short of happiness. However you choose to spend your money in retirement, getting more and better things will not deliver you the good life you expect.

The minimalist movement does touch on something important: your possessions will not make you happy. In my opinion, it also misses something important. While minimalists identify the problem, getting rid of your possessions and simplifying your life doesn't provide all the answers. Yes, experiences and freedom might have advantages over accumulating possessions, but they have their own problems. The Christian answer is that we were made to bring glory to our Father in Heaven. As Blaise Pascal famously put it, we all have a God-shaped vacuum inside us that nothing else can fill. If we seek happiness in our retirement years from possessions or experiences, we will be disappointed. A life actively serving Jesus will be a happier life than one spent serving only yourself.

Don't be dominated by the idea of leaving a legacy

When the end of your life looms large in your thinking, some people look to establish something that will outlast them. This could be a scholarship to be given annually in their name or a donation to some organisation that will record it on a plaque in their meeting room. There are too many churches that entertain this urge for a legacy as well, with previous members having their names attached to pews to recognise large donations they have made.

The desire to have ourselves remembered by others after we die is ultimately a selfish ambition. If we have departed this life, what does it matter if those who remain remember us in ten or a hundred years' time? The drive to have our name remembered is just one another way we think too highly of ourselves. Our self-worth comes from being children of God. That is the legacy we should be concerned with leaving: that Jesus be glorified.

We should again look to examples of those who have gone before us. Moses was humble[9] and made no effort for others to memorialise him. John the Baptist, the enormously popular and important prophet, stated that he was happy for Jesus to increase while he decreased.[10] A great many people who did great work for God in the Bible are never named.[11] John Calvin, the great Reformer, instructed others to bury him in an unmarked grave so that others could not go on pilgrimages to it. The desire for a lasting legacy can take the focus off Jesus and onto ourselves.

It is undoubtedly true what the Teacher of Ecclesiastes says:

> *For of the wise as of the fool there is no enduring remembrance, seeing that in the days to come all will have been long forgotten. How the wise dies just like the fool!*
>
> (Ecclesiastes 2:16)

When you are gone, people will forget you. In a relatively short time, no one alive will remember most of us. And that is perfectly OK. Our hope for the future is eternal life, not having things named after ourselves. If we are forgotten by the living, but remembered by our God, that is a great outcome!

There is another danger with seeking to be remembered: we may end up using our money with mixed motives. If we establish a scholarship in our own name, that may end up doing much good for the world. However, the money we give for that purpose is not purely given to help others; it is also given so others will remember us. We are all naturally selfish people. This could mean that we are not giving money to the best cause but to the cause that promotes our own glory. This is a great danger.

Jesus himself teaches us a better way:

> ²Thus, when you give to the needy, sound no trumpet before you, as the hypocrites do in the synagogues and in the streets, that they may be praised by others. Truly, I say to you, they have received their reward. ³But when you give to the needy, do not let your left hand know what your right hand is doing, ⁴so that your giving may be in secret. And your Father who sees in secret will reward you.
>
> *(Matthew 6:2-4)*

Be discreet; whatever you give, do your best to make sure it cannot be linked back to you. In that way, you remove the temptation of mixed motives that can arise from charitable donations. I know of secret donations of hundreds of thousands of dollars to theological colleges and church building funds. My own internship at my church was paid for mainly by a large anonymous donation. If God has blessed you with money, and you desire to use it well for his glory, look for a secret way to do this.

You should consider, especially in older age, how you can use your assets to serve God. That is a concept that too few people consider. Many people die, leaving much wealth behind, and it is quite possible that their children are comfortable and do not need a large inheritance. Have you considered using your will to support ministry and mission work? Some churches have been able to expand or purchase property due to former members' generosity through their estates. There are ways this kind of donation can also be kept relatively secret; speak to your accountant or church treasurer in confidence if this is something you would like to pursue.

But what if I don't have enough money in retirement?

Not everyone who retires will be wealthy; many retire and live on a very tight budget. If that's you, money is still something that can dominate your thinking and your life. After all, it is not money that is the root of all evil; it is the love of money that is the root of all evil.[12] If you don't have much money, but you spend a great deal of time and effort worrying about money, it still has a grip on your heart.

Remember that retirement as an expectation of a long holiday at the end of your life is a very new idea. If you don't have enough money to live for a long time without working, consider working part-time. It is not somehow failing at retirement to still be working; it might be a good thing for your mental health and social life. Don't be bitter that your retirement might not include too many cruise ships and new cars; that's the case for most people. You need to decide the most responsible way to serve Jesus in the situation you are in, and to work on trusting God's promises to meet all our needs.[13]

Where your treasure is, there your heart will be also

Peer pressure is a reality for retirees, not just for teenagers. Your next-door neighbours might have bought that new four-wheel drive and recently returned from that cruise through Europe. That exclusive golf club might count your former workmates as members. It is not easy to live differently from others around us. A retirement where you carefully use your money to support the gospel and you live a more modest life instead of a self-indulgent one will be weird to most people.

When the lure of fitting in and looking good becomes difficult to resist, remember this: money and possessions will never truly make you happy. Money is a good servant and a poor master. If you live for the next big thing, whether purchase or experience, there will always be something else. You will live in an endless cycle of greed and fear that others have things you do not have. Once money grips your heart, you run a considerable danger of increasing your selfishness and drifting away from ministry and service.

A life spent serving Jesus is far superior to a life spent serving money. Paul can say that he has learned to be content no matter the circumstances.[14] If you are a Christian, your worth is that Jesus died for you. You are of infinite value. It doesn't matter if others have more than you do or if they have less. It doesn't matter if you don't own the latest gadget or if you cannot tick off some list of travel destinations. If you have Jesus, you have wealth beyond your understanding. You have something no one can take from you and a satisfaction in life that cannot be replicated by the next big thing.

If our real treasure is in heaven and not on earth, we will want to use our earthly resources to support gospel work as much as we are able. We should use our worldly wealth to help others hear about Jesus,[15] either through your local church or some wider parachurch ministry or mission. If God has blessed you with money, look for opportunities to use it in a way that has eternal benefits. Using our wealth only for ourselves misses the great opportunities for the gospel all around us that are worth far more. Be generous to gospel work with enthusiasm;[16] God loves a cheerful giver.[17]

We are dust, and to dust we will return.[18] You cannot take it with you. When you stand before God, it will make no difference if you were wealthy or poor in this life. What will matter is how you used what God gave to you. Use your money to serve God and not just yourself. If God has blessed you with significant wealth in your latter years, use it well for his glory. Don't live like those who don't know Jesus and have no other option but to spend their retirement in self-indulgent luxury. If that's all we do with our money, that would be a sad response to Jesus indeed.

Chapter 12
Retirees in the church family

Older Christians can sometimes feel like second-class citizens in a local church. There are usually ministries aimed at children and teenagers and young adults. So many resources are poured into families with young children and university students. Seeing this emphasis can make older believers feel they are not a high priority in the church family.

On the other hand, some older Christians intentionally step back from service after retirement. I have heard several former elders and ministry leaders from a range of churches tell me that they have done their time, and now it is time for the younger ones to take their turn. This attitude of withdrawal says a great deal; it reveals that the common secular view of retirement as an extended holiday has crept into the thinking of even mature believers.

If older saints step back from active service in the local church, everyone loses. Everyone. The younger ones lose out from being built up by the retiree's experience and gifts, and the retiree themselves will run the real danger of growing more selfish and isolated from the body of Christ.

There is a better way. If retirees are intentional in their service in the local church, it unlocks huge benefits. Older believers have a lot to offer the local church.

Mentoring younger believers

Many churches start to divide their people into groups based on age. The teenagers attend the youth group, the young adults have their own Bible study, and perhaps there is a group for seniors. One problem with partitioning out the church into demographic segments is that older Christians often have very little interaction with younger Christians. It is more than possible for a young adult in a local church to never have had a conversation with a retiree who attends the same service on Sundays!

The first-century church didn't split things up quite so neatly. The apostles do give different instructions to various groups in the local churches, but it is obvious these groups mingled with one another. For example, we read this in Titus:

> *¹But as for you, teach what accords with sound doctrine. ²Older men are to be sober-minded, dignified, self-controlled, sound in faith, in love, and in steadfastness. ³Older women likewise are to be reverent in behavior, not slanderers or slaves to much wine. They are to teach what is good, ⁴and so train the young women to love their husbands and children, ⁵to be self-controlled, pure, working at home, kind, and submissive to their own husbands, that the word of God may not be reviled. ⁶Likewise, urge the younger men to be self-controlled. ⁷Show yourself in all respects to be a model of good works, and in your teaching show integrity, dignity, ⁸and sound speech that cannot be condemned, so that an opponent may be put to shame, having nothing evil to say about us.*
>
> *(Titus 2:1-8)*

This is part of a personal letter to Titus giving him instructions on what to teach the churches in Crete. Titus himself had a responsibility to teach everyone in the churches. He was to be such a good example that no one could say anything evil about him (v7-8).

The instructions to older men and older women emphasize the importance of their example in the church community. They were to model what it looks like to follow Jesus, not giving into the temptations inherent in each gender (v2-3). For such modelling to be seen by others, there must have been more interaction between generations than we see in many modern churches. Younger Christians had ready examples all around them of what self-control looked like; they just needed to look at and get to know some of the older people.

When Paul speaks about the older women, he specifically asks that they teach and train women younger than themselves (v3-4). This is more than simply imparting information like a teacher in a classroom might. This is about instructing the younger women in life. In the first century, when arranged marriages were the norm, almost all women would be married young. They would need help in knowing how to love their husbands and look after their households. The natural place to find this help is in the older women who have learnt all this through experience.

The same principle applies in the modern church. Where will newly married Christian women look for advice? Today, perhaps the first thing to occur to them would be an online forum, a self-help book, or a mother's group. While these resources might be helpful, the best Christian advice should be found among the older women within their local church.

Of course, the training of the younger believers by the older ones is not limited to marriage! Our modern cultures, which are not usually dominated by arranged marriages, have many single adults. Older Christian singles are in a good position to help the younger ones navigate a world where many are married and they are not. Likewise, believers experiencing the challenges of starting out in the workplace have many in their local church with decades of experience of being Christian in a secular workplace. Whatever new experience younger Christians encounter, it is very likely that someone older in the local church has the experience and maturity to help them process it and deal with the challenge in a godly way.

How might you be a help to the younger ones in your church? There are lots of options, both formal and informal.

The formal instruction of the younger believers in a church by the older ones can take a few different forms. In response to Titus 2, some churches have set up a formal one-to-one mentorship structure as a key ministry of the church. Older Christians are paired with new Christians or young adults to read the Bible, talk and pray. This helps relationships form that might otherwise not happen naturally, and both parties will benefit. Women's groups have also been helpful for this purpose, assuming that the groups attract those from a range of ages. Children's ministries and youth groups also offer an opportunity to get to know and teach the younger generations.

One of the most natural ways to encourage interaction between older and younger people in a local church is to eliminate most demographic-based Bible study groups. If a group contains both older and younger people, the range of perspectives will be a blessing for all who come. While a group made up of solely young adults might be exciting, with everyone having a lot in common, they need to hear from those with age and experience as well.

It doesn't have to be formal, however; there are all kinds of opportunities for older saints to teach and train the younger ones. It starts with building relationships. Next Sunday, intentionally seek out a younger person you don't know well and talk to them. In my experience, it is not only younger people who stick together in the local church; older people also stick with older people! If both sides break out of their comfort zone, relationships will start to form across generations. That way, when a younger believer has a problem to solve, they already have a network of older Christians they know and trust to talk to. This cannot help but strengthen a church family.

I need to include a word of caution here. Even if you are an older, mature Christian with much to offer, you don't know everything. You need to work at humility, even if you are mentoring younger believers. The advice you offer might simply be based on your experience and not on clear Bible teaching; sometimes it is hard to tell the difference. We must not be domineering of others in our attempt to be an encouragement. It is also possible that younger people might choose not to take our advice. Remember, the aim is to be an encouragement and source of help; you want to point people to Jesus and not have them idolise you.

Consider service in a leadership position

Almost every church I know of struggles to recruit

enough elders and deacons. Those in their 40s and 50s might well be faithful people, but they are also busy people. They are at the peak of their careers and are often raising children at the same time. Those who are retired can often be away on holidays for long stretches and unwilling to serve in a way that requires significant commitment.

The word 'elder' naturally refers to those who are older in age. The elders of tribes in the Old Testament would naturally be the older ones in the family. Most people in church leadership positions will naturally be older rather than younger. This doesn't mean that all elders need to be old; the example of Timothy shows us that age should not be the main determining factor of who is suitable to be in church leadership.[1]

Age does, however, bring advantages. Those who have been in the church for a long time have had the opportunity to deepen their knowledge. Even if you don't feel you know very much, being in a good church for decades provides a solid foundation for your faith. Most retirees in the church probably have a more robust Bible knowledge and theology than most new Christians. In a world where Bible knowledge is generally weak, you likely have a great deal to offer.

In addition, having life experience matters. Church leaders often have to make practical decisions about people and church programs. It is a great help in the leadership team to have people with life experience to help with such decisions.

Another great blessing that retired Christians in the church have is time. All of us have many responsibilities every week, but most retirees have more control over how they plan their week. If you could use that time to make a real difference to the local church, I would argue that is one of the best things you could do to fill your week!

When I first started pastoral ministry in my late 20s, I had one elder serving alongside me who was retired. My fellow elder was a godly man who had time to accompany me on visits, to thoughtfully consider whatever issues we faced, and to pray. He prevented me from making some rash decisions and encouraged me. I will always be grateful for his help in many ways. Here was a man who used his retirement well, and the local church was much stronger for his service.

If you are going to retire soon or have recently retired, I urge you to consider if you can use your experience and time to serve the church in some leadership position. It could be helping with the children's ministry; it could be volunteering with administration; it could be training to become an elder or a deacon. It is too easy to fill your week with recreational activities and leave a vacuum in the local church. Be a contributor and not just a consumer.

There is great benefit in being a faithful church member

If the last section made you break out in a cold sweat, don't worry; you don't need to be an elder to serve well in the local church. Faithful, consistent service as an ordinary church member is worth more than many give it credit for.

All Christians have spiritual gifts and are to use them to build up the church family.[2] That might be in leadership, but it might also be in other ways. Coming to church week by week and actively welcoming visitors will have a significant impact. Attending a Bible study group and helping others to understand and apply God's word has real value. Spending time talking and getting to know others encourages your church family as well.

The key is commitment and consistency. The local church is not supposed to be like a movie theatre, where all present come for the show but have no intention of interacting with one another. The local church is more like a family. Coming to church week on week with an attitude of welcome and service greatly encourages others.

An older lady I know struggles with all kinds of health problems. Just getting through the day and the week is hard for her. Yet, faithfully, Sunday by Sunday, she comes to church. She smiles and is genuinely happy at what God has done for her in Jesus. Coming to church is a significant effort for her. Those who don't know her well are unaware of just how significant, for she doesn't broadcast it. I see in her simple, consistent example that the local church matters to her and that she loves her church family.

You can teach an old dog new tricks

It is possible for someone to be in a local church with solid Bible teaching for decades without learning all that much. I know that sounds strange, but it is true. We don't learn by osmosis. We don't increase our Bible knowledge by simply being in the same room as good Bible teaching. We need to reflect on it day and night, talk about it, read further and pray about it.

When we are working or raising a family, sometimes we don't have the time or emotional energy to make the most of the local church's teaching opportunities. Workers might skip extra seminars when they are offered and fail to engage regularly with Bible study groups. Retirees have the time to engage more deeply with the teaching that is provided; make the most of this opportunity.

You are never too old to learn. There are all kinds of opportunities for deepening your knowledge of God through his Word in the local church. Join a Bible study group. Attend optional seminars and conventions offered in your city. Read books on the same topic being covered at church; work hard to make the most of the Scriptures. Even those who are older should be seeking to adjust their opinions and worldview when exposed to the Word of God. All of us can grow in our understanding and strive to become more like Jesus.

I have known several retirees who have decided to go further than this and enrol part-time in a local theological college. Some colleges offer evening courses or extension seminars. Even if you have no intention of serving in pastoral ministry, this is a good opportunity to learn more about life with our great God.

The church family helps deal with loneliness

Many older people find their world has shrunk from what it used to be. They have fewer social interactions than before, not having a workplace to go to day by day. Some older people have never married or have outlived their spouse, living alone and only seeing other people when shopping or on errands. Loneliness is becoming an epidemic in many countries. Some older friends of mine have commented that much of their social life revolves around attending medical appointments and funerals!

This is another great benefit of being an active part of a local church: you have a ready-made family who cares for you. Even if you don't have physical family members who live nearby, there is a whole community of people who love you. They should notice when you don't make it to church.

So many non-Christian people, in comparison, have a very small social circle. You notice this most often at funerals. Many people have funerals attended only by immediate family and a few close friends. In contrast, many Christian funerals are quite large. Many people will know you if you are part of a church.

Other ways of increasing social interaction often don't lead to the depth of relationship you can find in the local church. Book clubs and cycling groups do encourage mingling, and attending the local gym might mean you make a few friends. Compared to these clubs, the local church provides a much closer connection to one another because of Jesus. You have people who genuinely care for you even though you might have nothing else in common. There is something special about the church that you cannot find anywhere else.

There are opportunities to minister to other older people

Throughout this book, I have advocated for churches

and ministries to have people of different ages mingling as much as possible. There are, however, unique ministry opportunities that retirees have in the local church that others might find more difficult to serve in.

Retirement can be difficult. Transitioning to retirement might lead people to feel aimless and even depressed. If you have been through that before, you are in a great position to help others who go through this after you. Keep an eye out for those around you in that position. Make a time to talk over coffee; you might be a great blessing to someone whose retirement expectations might not be being met.

The truth is that many older people in our society would love more social contact; they may also be more interested in spiritual matters than they once were. When representatives from local churches visit people in aged care facilities, they generally get a positive reception from staff and residents. Perhaps you could visit people in your local nursing home regularly? Perhaps you could help transport older people to church services or just call them to see how they are? Your kindness in this kind of simple ministry might end up with eternal consequences for that person.

More churches would benefit from thinking strategically about how to minister to older people. Most churches do run youth groups and children's ministries, which, of course, have great value for the gospel. We must not forget the older saints in our midst and consider how to reach non-Christian older people with the gospel. Older believers in the local church need teaching and encouragement. They need fellowship. They need to be challenged to resist temptation and serve Jesus. I know of one church that employed an older man to co-ordinate a pastoral visitation and Bible study plan for the retirees in the church. You don't need to be on the church staff to do this, though! If you stop and think about it, there is always some way you can encourage other older people in your church. You could meet a single person for a regular cup of coffee. You could make a point of visiting those in hospital or calling up those who have long-term illnesses that prevent them from coming to church services.

The local church is such a central place to both serve and be served, and this is especially true for older people. Don't step back from service or think that all important ministry is done by or for young people. Your involvement in the local church is critical. Others need your gifts. Your experience and the time you have at your disposal can be well used to further the kingdom of God.

Chapter 13
Being salt and light as a retiree

Once someone becomes a Christian, everything changes. They start doing things they had no interest in before, like going to church and reading the Bible. They stop doing things that they used to love, perhaps including heavy drinking and gambling. It is like a new birth; everything about life is now seen through a different lens. While all of these changes are wonderful, there can be an unhelpful side effect. It is more than possible that the new convert starts to lose their non-Christian friends.

This happens to so many Christians. After the Spirit has changed their life in so many ways, they stop wanting to live the same way their friends do. Their friends might also find them odd. Without consciously deciding to do so, the Christian starts to drift off and spend all of their social time with other Christians. It is far more comfortable to be with those who share your love for Jesus and your passion for the Bible.

If we fast forward to the retirement years, most Christians have been in the church for a long time. Besides a few neighbours or family members, it is likely that all of their social circle are also Christians. While this is perfectly understandable, I think it is essential for us to lift our eyes to see the opportunities God gives us in a world dominated by non-Christians. We cannot remain only in our 'holy huddle'; we need to be making an impact on the world.

Salt and light always have an impact

Jesus made it clear that he intended for his disciples to influence the world around them, saying:

> [13]*"You are the salt of the earth, but if salt has lost its taste, how shall its saltiness be restored? It is*

no longer good for anything except to be thrown out and trampled under people's feet. ¹⁴You are the light of the world. A city set on a hill cannot be hidden. ¹⁵Nor do people light a lamp and put it under a basket, but on a stand, and it gives light to all in the house. ¹⁶In the same way, let your light shine before others, so that they may see your good works and give glory to your Father who is in heaven."

(Matthew 5:13-16)

What do salt and light have in common? Why has Jesus put them together here? It has to do with influence. A small amount of salt influences the whole dish; you notice when someone has added a pinch of salt to a stew. A small amount of light influences the entire room; even one candle added to a previously dark room means people can see. Christians should be like this in the broader world. Even if there are only a small number of Christians in a society, the whole society should be better because of those few believers' influence.

We can go further than 'should'. Jesus' language is very strong in Matthew 5. When he speaks of salt losing its taste in v13, he doesn't mean that salt degrades over time. No, salt is always salty. If it is not salty, it is not salt at all. Jesus' point is that Christians are salt; we cannot help having an influence on the world around us. We should be useful. We see the same idea in v15 when it comes to light. We don't want to hide away from the world where we have little influence; we need to live in full view of the world around us. If those who are not Christian are to one day give glory to our Father in heaven, they will need to meet and be influenced by Christians in some way.

All of this brings us back to retirement. The most comfortable option for Christian retirees is to spend all of their social time and service in the local church or with Christian friends. The problem is that most of us live in societies where the vast majority of people care nothing for Jesus.[1] Staying where it is comfortable for us means we are not living as Jesus calls us to in Matthew 5. We need to be more thoughtful about how to influence the world around us.

I know, I know; it's a massive task for a small number of Christians to influence a big world that is often hostile to Christianity. But isn't that what Jesus envisaged in Matthew 5? You don't need a lot of salt to improve a bland dish or a lot of light to make a dark room easy to walk through. If all the Christian people lived faithful, helpful lives in their local communities, the world would be a better place. We need a bigger vision than a retirement spent in our 'holy huddle'.

Engaging with your local community

God has placed each of us in a local community. This is a great place to start connecting with the non-Christian world. Get to know your neighbours; stop for a chat when you see them near the postbox or invite them over for a cup of tea. You will likely see one another incidentally as you go through your week, so go out of your way to be friendly and helpful. Anyone can do this. You don't need to be an extrovert or a people person; start by getting to know one or two people who live near you.

If your social life mainly revolves around other Christians and your church, you will need to be intentional about broadening your horizons. Make an effort to maintain contact with old work friends. Look at the social groups in your area that are based around activities you already enjoy. Many older people choose to join secular community groups, forcing them to mingle with a broader range of people than they usually do. You will find that not only do you bring a Christian influence into the group you join, but you will also benefit and grow from the friendship of others and find opportunities to share the gospel at the same time.

All Christians need to have contact with non-Christians. As a pastor in a local church, I always run the risk of spending 100% of my time with Christians. I have joined a local golf club that matches me up with random strangers every time I play to counter this. While this puts me outside my comfort zone socially, it does give me opportunities I would not otherwise have to get to know non-Christian people. Whether you are into golf, swimming, chess or food, there is bound to be some opportunity to mingle with people interested in the same thing. You can indulge your hobbies while also intentionally creating friendships with non-Christian people with an aim to creating evangelistic opportunities.

If you live in a retirement village or an aged care facility, you have even more opportunities to be salt and light in a dark world. There are many social events organised in these communities and some even have shared meals several times a day. You cannot help but build friendships in such an environment. Look to be a positive influence on those around you; don't just fall into the trap of complaining or negativity. Over time, when the big issues of life arise in your new friends' lives, you can naturally give your opinion as a Christian. You never know what opportunities God might give you in that context.

Another possible way to be involved in the wider unbelieving world is to volunteer. Many organisations look for help from community members, with retirees being one of the most active groups. You could give some time to a charity shop or be trained to help teach English to migrants. You could mentor children at the local primary school or join the local Rotary club in their efforts. All of these options put you into contact with non-Christians you would not otherwise meet. Don't put your lamp under a basket. Intentionally look for places you can have an influence.

Not all of our interactions with the secular world around us need to be explicitly evangelistic, even though we should remain aware of opportunities to share the gospel all the time. It is valid to volunteer for a good cause alongside those who are not Christians. This could mean helping at a soup kitchen or fundraising for charity. It could be joining a local men's shed to help make toys and wheelchairs for those in developing countries. Our local communities should be better in all kinds of ways because Christians are an active part of them.

Evangelism as a lifestyle

Jesus told his disciples to make disciples of all nations.[2] Paul told the church in Rome that it was critical to speak the gospel to people in order for them to be saved.[3] Elsewhere, he told his readers that he strived creatively to do all he could to save even some for Jesus.[4] All Christians should be involved in speaking about Jesus in some way.

What would that look like for a retiree? Extra time is one big advantage those who are retired have when it comes to evangelism. Retirees can cultivate friendships with more regular catch-ups. A combination of time and social opportunities means extra opportunities to talk about the hope that we have.

A friend of mine who was in his seventies had always been a passionate evangelist throughout his life and thought strategically about how he could use his retirement for the sake of the gospel. He had moved into a retirement village with his wife. He intentionally purchased the newspaper and a coffee from the same local stores in order to build up friendships with the staff. He took up chess to take part in regular games with other residents of his retirement village. This man prayed daily, by name, for these store owners and chess opponents, and then looked for opportunities to talk about Jesus. None of this is beyond most Christians. We just need to lift our eyes to see that the fields are ripe for harvest.

When we are older, our friends also tend to be older. They also have the time to think about big issues that they may have been avoiding for many years. As they attend funerals or perhaps come to terms with their own mortality, there might be opportunities to share the gospel that we would never have imagined earlier in life. Older people need Jesus as much as younger people do. We need to make the most of the time and opportunities God gives to us.

You don't need to be a full-time evangelist

Perhaps the previous section scares you; most of us don't think of ourselves as natural evangelists. While it is inspiring to see how many others have intentionally built evangelism into their lives, the whole idea might be terrifying for some of us. Don't worry; even if you are not an outgoing person, you can have a significant impact on those around you.

Christians are called to be different to the world around us. And, in many ways, most Christians do stand out. Even in difficult times, we have hope because we know Jesus is King and the future is secure. Christians are usually far more generous with their money and more committed to the church than others are to any community they are part of.

Sometimes we don't realise how different our worldview is from the broader culture because most of our friends share our Christian convictions. But if we intentionally expand our social group to include more non-Christian people, our different way of living and thinking should stand out. To use Peter's language, we should aim to live such good lives that those around us notice it and end up worshipping God in time for the Last Day.[5]

All of this means that you don't have to constantly talk about Jesus when you have contact with non-Christian people. That is pretty artificial anyway; they will know you are only considering them as some kind of target rather than trying to build genuine friendships. The apostle Peter envisaged those in our world seeing Christ in our lives; that will not happen if we don't know any non-Christian people! As you live life together with those in our world, they will notice the different way you see things. This might lead to questions and opportunities for the gospel that arise naturally rather than forcing the conversation in a gospel direction.

Use your influence with your children and grandchildren well

All families are different, and not all retirees will have children or grandchildren. If you have been blessed in this way, you have a ready-built way to make a significant difference in others' lives.

Many retirees help their children by looking after their grandchildren every week. This can feel like a burden, and perhaps sometimes it will be! It also provides an opportunity on a few different fronts. You can build deeper relationships with your children. You can become close to your grandchildren and create a connection that will last for the rest of your life. And, as many have told me, it makes you feel young to spend time at the park and to play with Lego again!

As Christians, our faith should mean that we look for more than building better relationships with our family members; even non-Christians do that! We need to aim higher. We want to be a positive influence on our family members for the gospel.

I know of several retired couples whose children are not believers. They are upset that their children don't share their faith and don't raise their own children to know Jesus. They have realised, however, that being a grandparent gives you a significant influence in the lives of your grandchildren. When you look after your grandchildren, you can read the Bible to them, sing

Christian songs with them, or even bring them along with you to church.[6] You might well be the only way they will hear about Jesus, so use your influence well.

Many parents and grandparents are persistent in prayer for their children and grandchildren. It is heartbreaking when a child you raised to love the Lord turns away; there is no guarantee this is forever. Keep praying. Keep looking for opportunities. I know of several people who credit the influence of a faithful, praying grandmother as a critical factor in their conversion many years later.

Whatever your stage in life, all Christians have a responsibility to actively be part of the wider world. We must resist the urge to withdraw into our local churches and ignore our neighbours. God has placed us where we are for a reason. Open your eyes and think intentionally about the opportunities to get to know non-Christian people near where you live, in your family, or in interest groups you might join. Who knows? Your presence in the lives of those around you might make an eternal difference to someone.

Closing challenge:
An intentionally God-glorifying retirement

Our culture has a very clear idea of what the latter years of our lives should ideally look like. We should retire from work as early as possible and then indulge ourselves in recreation for as long as possible. That sounds like a great idea to most of us because we have been trained to expect it. We have been told that this is what we are entitled to as our right. We likely know people who spend months travelling each year before going back to their beautiful home in their shiny new car.

The reality is not as rosy as the advertisements promise. Relationship breakdowns, a lack of motivation and purpose, and increased health problems are all common in the retirement years. As death gets closer, the big issues of life start to make us think more deeply. Is this all there is? The truth is that we were meant for more than a lengthy holiday. God created us to glorify him. Jesus died for us to give us new life and purpose and to serve him well. The Spirit empowers us to live a godly life. Too often, Christians put God to the side and live just like those who don't know Jesus. We need to be far more intentional than that.

When we open the pages of the Bible, we see that God has told us a lot about old age. We see direct instruction about respecting older people. We are reminded that old age is a blessing from God and not a curse, not something to be ashamed of or avoided. God, in his kindness, also shows us many examples of people who honoured God well in their later years, as well as cautionary tales of those who lived those last years badly. The Bible is a book that shows the troubles and limitations of old age but doesn't describe those who are older as in any way inferior to the young and the healthy.

Retirees are uniquely placed to use the experience and extra time they have at their disposal to serve Jesus. The local church needs older people to serve in all kinds of ways, from leadership positions through to hospitality. The local church can be a help to retirees who need assistance or who struggle with loneliness, and retirees can be a great help to younger people with their encouragement and wisdom. On top of this, older believers have many ready-made opportunities in their local communities to make the world a better place, even to help point other people towards Jesus.

Retirement doesn't need to be the selfish extended holiday many expect it to be. It can be a time of real Christian growth, the use of the experience and gifts God gave you, and a strong finish to a faithful life. Don't settle for what the world promises in retirement. Serve Jesus well.

Acknowledgements

Firstly, I would like to thank God. He has been kind to me in so many ways that I do not deserve. I face the future, including any future retirement period, with confidence because of what Jesus has done for me.

I would like to thank my wife Andrea who is a constant help and support to me. Her wise advice and thoughtful outlook on life, including on this topic, have helped sharpen my thinking. And her editing of the manuscript often helped me express myself more clearly and helpfully.

My two early reviewers, The Right Reverend Dr Peter Brain and Reverend Dr Stephen Rarig, have been generous with their time, experience and advice. Each of them kindly took the time to give feedback on an earlier version of this manuscript, and this is a better book because of their input.

Thanks also to the congregation of All Nations Presbyterian Church. This has been my church family for many years, and I have been greatly encouraged by the example of my brothers and sisters, including retirees, as they seek to serve Jesus.

About the Author

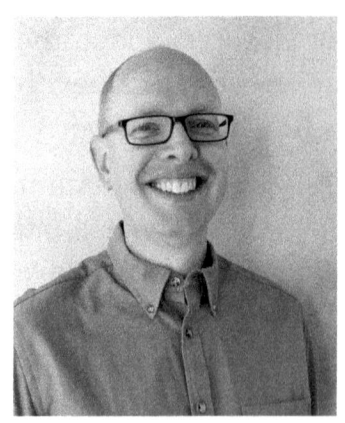

Simon van Bruchem is a pastor of All Nations Presbyterian Church in Perth, Western Australia, where he has served since 2007. He completed his Master of Divinity at Trinity Theological College after a previous career as an industrial chemist. He considers it a great privilege to be able to study and teach the wonderful news about Jesus from the Bible full time.

Simon is married to Andrea, and together they parent three boys, ensuring life is consistently interesting and busy. When he is not involved with his work of pastoring the church and his family, he loves to tend to his fruit trees, play golf and read widely.

Simon has also authored 'Fear Not: What the Bible has to say about angels, demons, the occult and Satan'.

Simon blogs regularly at
www.writtenforourinstruction.com

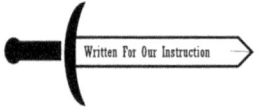

Endnotes

Introduction

[1] Milne, D. 2013, *The Psychology of Retirement*, Wiley-Blackwell, p25.

[2] One example is David C. Borchard 2008, *The Joy of Retirement: Finding Happiness, Freedom, and the Life You've Always Wanted*, Harper Collins Focus, Nashville.

[3] Matthew 5:14-16.

[4] Matthew 10:38.

[5] Romans 12:1-2.

Chapter 1 A history lesson: how did we get here?

[1] President Macron proposed increasing the retirement age in France from 62 to 64, then retracted this due to countrywide protests. https://www.nytimes.com/2020/01/11/world/europe/france-pension-protests.html (accessed 17 January 2021).

[2] President Berlusconi faced a financial crisis in 2003 and proposed relaxing the generous pension system that permitted retirement as early as 57 for long-term government employees. The proposal was met with a major strike that crippled air travel and schools among other industries. https://www.theguardian.com/world/2003/oct/24/italy (accessed 19 January 2021).

[3] Numbers 8:24-26. Note also that Zechariah the priest in Luke 1:18-25 was elderly but was still in active service in the temple.

[4] Milne, D. 2013, *The Psychology of Retirement*, Wiley-Blackwell, p3.

[5] Milne, D. 2013, *The Psychology of Retirement*, Wiley-Blackwell, p3.

[6] von Herbay, Axel, Feb 2014 *Otto Von Bismarck Is Not the Origin of Old Age at 65*, The Gerontologist, Volume 54, Issue 1, Page 5.

[7] For a humorous overview of the history of retirement, consider https://www.nytimes.com/1999/03/21/jobs/the-history-of-retirement-from-early-man-to-aarp.html (accessed 5 October 2020).

[8] Housel, Morgan 2020 *The Psychology of Money: Timeless Lessons on Wealth, Greed and Happiness*, narrated by Chris Hill, Harriman House, Introduction, audiobook.

[9] Keller, Timothy 2016, *Making Sense of God: An Invitation to the Sceptical*, Hodder & Stoughton, London, p13.

Chapter 2 What makes your life worthwhile?

[1] This is not a book about psychology, and I am not a psychologist. If you are interested in knowing more about the impact of retirement on wellbeing, Derek Milne's book *The Psychology of Retirement* (Wiley-Blackwell, 2013) is an accessible place to start.

[2] Genesis 1:28.

[3] John 5:17.

[4] Genesis 1:26-28.

[5] Such as Cain and Abel, Genesis 4:2.

[6] Such as David who was a shepherd (1 Samuel 16:11) and Gideon who laboured as he did due to the oppression by foreign invaders in Judges 6:11.

[7] Unless specified, all Bible references in this book are from the ESV Bible (Holy Bible English Standard Version), copyright ©2001 by Crossway, a publishing ministry of Good News Publishers. Used by permission. All rights reserved.

[8] Martin Luther's tract *'The Priesthood of all Believers'* summarises this doctrine well.

[9] Romans 1:23.

[10] Ecclesiastes 2:23.

[11] Ecclesiastes 2:24 notes that this is a gift from God.

[12] This is particularly a problem for retired pastors. Pastors get accustomed to a high level of respect within the church family, and when they no longer have the formal role that is linked to that respect, they have to adjust to being a regular part of a church community. This can lead to bitterness or depression, or worse undermining the current pastor in an attempt to stay important in the eyes of the congregation.

[13] Romans 3:24.

[14] Romans 8:38-39.

[15] Romans 8:14.

[16] Hebrews 12:23.

[17] John 3:16.

[18] John 10:10.

[19] 1 Timothy 4:8.

[20] Ephesians 2:8.

[21] Philippians 3:7, 1 Corinthians 1:31.

[22] James 2:18.

[23] Ephesians 2:10.

[24] 1 Corinthians 8:11.

Chapter 3 Doing nothing can kill you; the need for purpose

[1] Milne, D. 2013, *The Psychology of Retirement*, Wiley-Blackwell, p53.

[2] Ecclesiastes 1:2-4.

[3] Ecclesiastes 2:11.

[4] Exodus 20:11, referring to Genesis 2:1-3.

[5] Deuteronomy 5:15.

[6] 2 Thessalonians 3:11.

[7] 1 Thessalonians 3:10.

[8] 1 Timothy 5:13.

[9] Quoted on https://money.cnn.com/2015/08/31/technology/minecraft-creator-tweets/index.html, accessed 9 December 2020.

[10] Keller, Timothy 2016, *Making Sense of God: An Invitation to the Sceptical,* Hodder & Stoughton, London, p57-76.

[11] Matthew 6:33.

[12] 1 Peter 2:12.

[13] 1 Timothy 4:7-8.

[14] John 10:10.

[15] Philippians 4:4, 10-13.

Chapter 4 Death sharpens the mind

[1] This idea is repeated in Ecclesiastes 3:13 and 22.

[2] You can also find the Teacher discuss the satisfaction of food in Ecclesiastes 9:7.

[3] Ecclesiastes 9:9.

[4] Ecclesiastes 11:7.

[5] Hebrews 9:27.

[6] Hebrews 9:27.

[7] This phrase is repeated often in Ecclesiastes, including in 1:14, 2:11 and 2:17.

[8] Genesis 1:1.

[9] Romans 1:21, Acts 17:27.

[10] Romans 3:1-20, Ephesians 2:1-3.

[11] Romans 3:21-26, Ephesians 2:4-6.

[12] Romans 8:1.

[13] 1 John 3:1.

[14] An example of this was King Omri in 1 Kings 16:15-28. The Bible tells us that he was popular with the people (v16), more powerful than his rivals (v22), and built a new capital city during his twelve year reign (v24). Yet God assessed Omri as evil in his sight for continuing in the worship of golden calves.

[15] For more exploration regarding what God assesses vs what we assess, visit https://writtenforourinstruction.com/assessing-the-right-things/.

[16] https://slate.com/culture/2011/11/bucket-list-what-s-the-origin-of-the-term.html, accessed 22 December 2020.

[17] Piper, John 2018 *Don't Waste Your Life*, Crossway Books, Wheaton, Illinois, p8.

[18] Ecclesiastes 7:2.

Chapter 5 Don't substitute 'retirement' for 'heaven'

[1] This can also be seen in Psalm 16:10-11, where David expresses his confidence that God will not abandon him after death but he will experience pleasures at God's right hand forevermore.

[2] 2 Samuel 12:23.

[3] This confidence in the future that the Old Testament believers had is well explained in the famous 'by faith' chapter in Hebrews 11.

[4] C.S. Lewis, 2013 *The Weight of Glory: A Collection of Lewis' Most Moving Addresses*, HarperCollins, London, p32.

[5] Romans 1:22-23.

[6] Matthew 6:25.

[7] Matthew 4:4, Deut 8:3.

[8] Think of songs like 'Swing Low, Sweet Chariot', for example.

[9] Deuteronomy 6:7-9.

[10] Psalm 1.

[11] John 3:16, 6:54.

[12] 1 Corinthians 13:12.

Chapter 6 Direct Biblical teaching on age and maturity

[1] Job 32:2.

[2] This is seen all through the Old Testament, including Exodus 4:29, Deuteronomy 19:12, and Ruth 4:11.

[3] Acts 6:1-6, 1 Timothy 5:3.

[4] 1 Timothy 4:12.

[5] Genesis 15:15.

[6] Genesis 25:7-8.

[7] Judges 8:32.

[8] 2 Chronicles 24:15.

[9] This can be seen in Deuteronomy 5:33 and 22:7.

[10] 1 Samuel 10:24, 1 Kings 1:25.

[11] Psalm 72:15.

[12] 1 Samuel 2:32.

[13] Proverbs 1:8.

[14] Proverbs 1:20, 2:1, 3:1.

[15] Proverbs 1:5.

[16] Proverbs 23:22.

[17] Lamentations 5:21, Ruth 4:11.

[18] 1 Timothy 5:1-2.

[19] Acts 6:1-6.

[20] 1 Timothy 5:9-10. Note also that the church was only to support widows who did not have their own families; if they had relatives, the care for the widow was to rest on the family (v16).

[21] John 19:26-27.

Chapter 7 Biblical examples

[1] 1 Corinthians 10:11 uses this phrase when applying the situation of the Israelites in the wilderness to Christians in first-century Greece.

[2] Genesis 12:4.

[3] Genesis 12:4, Genesis 15:6, Romans 4:3.

[4] God changed his name from Abram to Abraham in Genesis 17:5, which means 'the father of many nations'.

[5] Genesis 15:3.

[6] Genesis 17:17.

[7] Romans 4, Hebrews 11:18, James 2:21.

[8] Exodus 2:15.

[9] Exodus 3:11, 4:10, 4:13.

[10] Exodus 7:7.

[11] Deuteronomy 34:7.

[12] Hebrews 3:5.

[13] Numbers 12:3.

[14] 1 Corinthians 1:26-31, also a major theme in Hannah's song in 1 Samuel 1:7-8 and Mary's song in Luke 1:51-53.

[15] You can read the full story in Numbers 13.

[16] Joshua 14:10-11.

[17] Joshua 24:29.

[18] Samuel killed the king of the Amalekites by his own hand when Saul had not done what he was told to in 1 Samuel 15:32-33.

[19] 1 Samuel 8:1-2.

[20] John 13:23, 20:2

[21] Acts 3-4.

[22] Acts 8:14.

[23] Galatians 2:9.

[24] For example, see 1 John 2:1, 18, 28.

[25] 2 John 1, 3 John 1.

[26] You can read of this in 1 Kings 3.

[27] 1 Kings 3:16-28.

[28] 1 Kings 4:1-20.

[29] You can read this lengthy prayer in 1 Kings 8.

[30] 1 Kings 10:23-25.

[31] Solomon married Pharaoh's daughter, as we are told in 1 Kings 3:1.

[32] 2 Kings 16:3.

[33] 2 Kings 18:3.

[34] 2 Kings 19:1-7.

[35] Romans 12:15.

Chapter 8 Seeking the kingdom first in older age

[1] Matthew 22:37, quoting Deuteronomy 6:5.

[2] Matthew 22:39.

[3] Matthew 6:24.

[4] Ephesians 5:28.

[5] Matthew 18:8-9.

[6] Matthew 10:37.

[7] Revelation 2:10.

[8] 1 Kings 19:18.

[9] Psalm 90:2, Ephesians 5:16.

[10] Matthew 25:14-30.

[11] Matthew 25:21.

Chapter 9 Fighting the urge to criticise change and idolise the 'good old days'

[1] This is attributed to Socrates (ca. 425 BC). It first appeared in the Cambridge dissertation of Kenneth John Freeman in 1907, summarising a variety of

passages where Socrates and Plato expressed similar sentiments.

[2] Rosling, Hans with Rosling, Ola and Rosling Ronnlund, Anna 2008 *Factfulness: Ten Reasons We're Wrong About The World – And Why Things Are Better Than You Think*, Sceptre, London, audiobook.

[3] Exodus 2:23.

[4] Exodus 1:16.

[5] 2 Tim 3:14-17.

[6] Colossians 3:16.

[7] Psalm 1:2.

[8] Romans 12:2.

[9] I recognise that there are debates over head coverings in some contexts based on 1 Corinthians 11:6-7, but nothing is instructed regarding clothing except that we need to beware of vain external adornment (1 Peter 3:3-4).

[10] 1 Corinthians 9:22.

Chapter 10 Serving Jesus despite loss of energy, disability and other limitations

[1] 1 Kings 11:29

[2] 1 Kings 14:2.

[3] 1 Samuel 4:15-18.

[4] 1 Kings 15:23.

[5] In 2 Corinthians 11:6 Paul admits he is unskilled in speaking, and 2 Corinthians 10:1 implies he is accused of being bold only in his writing and yet humble in person.

[6] Philippians 4:11.

[7] Philippians 4:4.

[8] As David did in Psalm 8.

[9] As Paul says in Romans 8:37-39, nothing can separate us from the love of God in Christ Jesus our Lord. Not even old age or disability.

[10] Revelation 21:1-4 reminds us that in the new creation there will be no more pain or crying or mourning.

Chapter 11 Retirement and money

[1] Matthew 6:24.

[2] One major financial institution, AMP, quotes a typical figure of $993,473 (https://www.amp.com.au/retirement/prepare-to-retire/retirement-money-needs, accessed 6 March 2021).

[3] If you're not convinced this is true, look up https://howrichami.givingwhatwecan.org/how-rich-am-i. Most people who live in the Western world are far wealthier in global terms than they think they are.

[4] You can see this in the parable of the talents, found in Matthew 25:13-30.

[5] Psalm 50:10 says that God owns the cattle on a thousand hills. I am sure many farmers thought those cows belonged to them, but ultimately they all belonged to God.

[6] James 5:5.

[7] Mark 12:42-44.

[8] If you are new to the idea of minimalism, you might want to watch *'The Minimalists'* documentary on Netflix or read books and blogs by Joshua Becker or Leo Babuta.

[9] Numbers 12:3.

[10] John 3:30.

[11] For example, there are multiple men of God in 1 Kings who function as prophets, and many of those who planted churches in the New Testament (such as Rome) are unknown to us.

[12] 1 Timothy 6:10.

[13] Philippians 4:19.

[14] Philippians 4:12-13. Paul says he can do all things through him who strengthens me.

[15] Luke 16:9.

[16] Romans 12:8.

[17] 2 Corinthians 9:7.

[18] Ecclesiastes 3:20.

Chapter 12 Retirees in the church family

[1] 1 Timothy 4:12.

[2] 1 Corinthians 12:1-11.

Chapter 13 Being salt and light as a retiree

[1] Perth, Western Australia, where I live, is one of the most secular cities in a very secular country. Although many people tick 'Christian' on the census, less than 5% would attend church more than once a month. (The annual average is 8%, according to https://mccrindle.com.au/insights/blogarchive/church-attendance-in-australia-infographic/ accessed 22 July 2021, but that is skewed by Sydney which has a much higher church attendance than other major cities). There would likely be less than 1% of the wider population in a Bible teaching church (of any denomination from Pentecostal to Reformed) on any given Sunday.

[2] Matthew 28:16-20.

[3] Romans 10:13-17.

[4] 1 Corinthians 9:22.

[5] 1 Peter 2:12.

[6] Some Christian grandparents report that their unbelieving children prohibit them from reading the Bible to their grandchildren or from taking them to church. Even if this is the case, you can be a positive influence, praying and living a godly life before them. Who knows? One day the opportunity might arise, and you will then be in a good position to make the most of it to explain the reason for the hope that you have.

Lightning Source UK Ltd.
Milton Keynes UK
UKHW022240110123
415100UK00009B/95